EYE EXAMINATION
AND REFRACTION

Modern Optometry

SERIES EDITOR

R. FLETCHER

Eye Examination and Refraction

R.J. ALLEN
BSc, FBCO, DCLP, FAAO
Consultant Clinician, City University, London

R. FLETCHER
MScTech, FBCO, FBOA, HD, FSMC (Hons),
DOrth, DCLP, FAAO
Emeritus Professor, City University, London
Docent II, Kongsberg Inginør Høgskole,
Kongsberg, Norge

D.C. STILL
FSMC(Hons), FBOA
Optometrist in practice in Dorset

MODERN
OPTOMETRY

OXFORD

BLACKWELL SCIENTIFIC PUBLICATIONS

LONDON EDINBURGH BOSTON

MELBOURNE PARIS BERLIN VIENNA

© 1991 by R.J. Allen, R. Fletcher,
D.C. Still

Blackwell Scientific Publications
Editorial offices:
Osney Mead, Oxford OX2 0EL
25 John Street, London WC1N 2BL
23 Ainslie Place, Edinburgh EH3 6AJ
3 Cambridge Center, Cambridge,
  Massachussetts 02142,USA
54 University Street, Carlton
  Victoria 3053, Australia

Other editorial offices:
Arnette SA
2, rue Casimir-Delavigne
75006 Paris
France

Blackwell Wissenschaft
Meinekestrasse 4
D-1000 Berlin 15
West Germany

Blackwell MZV
Feldgasse 13
A-1238 Wien
Austria

First published 1991

Set by Times Graphics
Printed in Great Britain at the Alden Press, Oxford
and bound by Hartnolls Ltd,
Bodmin, Cornwall.

DISTRIBUTORS
  Marston Book Services Ltd
  PO Box 87
  Oxford OX2 0DT
  (*Orders*: Tel: 0865 791155
        Fax: 0865 791927
        Telex: 837515

USA
  Mosby-Year Book, Inc.
  11830 Westline Industrial Drive
  St Louis, Missouri 63146
  (*Orders*: Tel: (800) 633–6699)

Canada
  Mosby-Year Book, Inc
  5240 Finch Avenue East
  Scarborough, Ontario
  (*Orders*: Tel: (416) 298–1588)

Australia
  Blackwell Scientific Publications
  (Australia) Pty Ltd
  54 University Street,
  Carlton, Victoria 3053
  (*Orders*: Tel: (03) 347–0300)

British Library
Cataloguing in Publication Data

Allen, R. J.
    Eye examination and refraction.
    1.Man. Eyes. Refraction. Testing
  I. Title II. Fletcher, R. III. Still, D. C.
  617.755075

  ISBN 0–632–02866–1

Contents

Introduction

This book is intended primarily to help newcomers to the profession, particularly those needing to revise for professional examinations, which are essential to practise in the UK. Three experienced optometrists with very different backgrounds, representing different generations, have combined to write about this most basic aspect of optometry. The three sections of the book (Chapters 1–8, 9–16 and 17–19) are easily recognizable, with obvious overlapping of certain features and slight differences of approach which reflect the viewpoints of the authors. The final chapters concentrate on 'case studies' which illustrate much of the earlier text in a way that is seldom presented; in some ways, this provides 'instant experience' to the novice.

Others should find uses for the book; for instance undergraduates and those returning to optometric practice; trainee ophthalmologists and experienced practitioners who feel ready to review and to revise their own approaches may also benefit. The authors have recognized the limits likely to be experienced by readers, for whom time is short and access to textbooks and journals probably not as easy as they might wish. Hence the references given have been selective; they have been chiefly concentrated in the middle chapters and are usually such as might prompt study of an unusual approach or suggest a wider literature. Most readers should already possess their own notes or even books which cover the subject differently. A fresh outlook often helps, which is one object of the present small text. It can be used as a 'tutorial', in parts or as a whole. The questions provided may be useful for revision.

Acknowledgements

We wish to thank our families and several colleagues who have been supportive in the process of preparing this text. Although unnamed, they are likely to recognize this sincere appreciation.

Mr Richard Miles of Blackwell Scientific Publications has been a tower of strength to the book, as publisher.

Some of the figures are by courtesy of colleagues and firms, for which we are grateful.

The Editor of *The Optician* kindly agreed that some of the cases from his journal might be used, slightly modified.

Part I
Routines and Extra Tests

Chapter 1
An Eye Examination

The Association of Optometrists' booklet entitled *What is an eye examination?* answers the question with this definition:

'An eye examination is a clinical check on the function and activity of a person's eyes and can lead to the early detection, not only of eye diseases, but also of other diseases. This examination is undertaken by an ophthalmic optician (optometrist). These practitioners have been specifically trained to examine eyes, to recognise and refer for medical attention patients exhibiting signs of ocular abnormality, to test vision and, where necessary, to prescribe and dispense spectacles or contact lenses according to the patient's needs.'

This definition leaves out a few details, such as the provision of aids for patients with partial sight, the giving of advice concerning visual ergonomics (lighting, etc.) and the treatment of binocular vision anomalies. However, the above definition is basically sound, and is a reasonable codification to which optometrists can refer.

The British College of Optometrists, in its 'Code of Ethics and Guidelines for Professional Conduct' (sections 1.3.1 and 1.3.2) gives advice regarding the ideal content of a routine eye examination and these guidelines are, broadly, echoed in the leaflet *Guidance for Candidates, Supervisors and Examiners on the Professional Qualifying Examination.*

The aim of the optometrist in carrying out an eye examination should be to fulfill the legal and moral obligations involved, and to provide the patient with the best service available within the confines of professional ability. This will require different tests and methods of investigation according to the presenting problems but the basics of a routine eye examination should always be applied so as to provide the practitioner with a certain minimum level of information. This does not mean that every patient must undergo a specific routine, regardless of their needs. Indeed there is absolutely no point in, for example, checking the refractive status of a patient who was last examined only six months previously and has only attended for a visual field screening, ophthalmoscopy and tonometry.

This book is aimed primarily at pre-registration optometrists, offering a simple grounding in the rationale behind the routine examination of the eyes, with an eye on part of the Professional Qualifying Examinations (PQE) of the British College of Optometrists (BCO). It may also be of use to the qualified practitioner who wishes to reassess routines either for the purpose of change, or so as to be better informed when supervising a pre-registration student.

For most of this text, the author has assumed that the patient is mature enough to respond accurately to full routine eye examination. In the case of young children different systems and tactics have to be used, and it is outside the scope of this book to cover this area.

A patient is entitled to some explanation of the procedures carried out during the eye examination, and what they reveal. Usually this can be done directly, but on some occasions the explanation must be given via a relative or close friend of the patient.

There are some sections of the text in which a particular gender of patient has been assumed. The author hopes that this is not taken as a sexist stand on his part; it is most definitely not intended as such, and any offence so caused is unintentional. In general, the optometrist will be referred to as male, and the patient as female.

Chapter 2
Aims and Objectives

Because of their importance some of the aims and objectives of a routine eye examination will now be repeated.

Most patients attending for a routine eye examination are not in a position to be able to judge the professional competence of the optometrist; they have their own ideas as to what the examination should comprise but are unlikely to comment upon the absence of an expected procedure. This does not mean, however, that they have no expectations of the practitioner. In fact the patient has a legally established right to expect a certain minimum standard of performance from the optometrist. This is enshrined in the legislation covering the area of negligence, and the practitioner is thereby expected to perform in a manner befitting his professional qualifications and experience.

The aims of a routine eye examination are simple; to determine the problems from which the patient is suffering and to deal with them in an appropriate fashion.

The eye examination can have several objectives:
1 The provision of a professional health care service for the benefit of the patient.
2 The determination of a prescription for any required optical appliance.
3 The enhancement of the standing of the profession of optometry in general, and of the individual practitioner.
4 The provision of income for the practitioner and ancillary staff.
These frequently overlap. With the exception of the last category (that of income generation) frequently they complement one another.

It is important to perceive the routine examination of the eyes as an end in itself, not merely as leading to the supply of spectacles. This can only be achieved by allowing an optometrist professional freedom in terms of time allowed for an eye examination, and expecting and encouraging the highest standards. An adequate standard of equipment is essential to enable the optometrist to complete an adequate examination in a reasonable time.

Patients generally recognize the practitioner as an integral part of the community and environment. The optometrist who works within a department store or spectacle boutique will inevitably be regarded as a glorified salesperson rather than as a professional healthcare specialist, regardless of the care extended to the patient in the consulting room. Practising within such surroundings does nothing to help the public appreciate the professional and clinical background of optometry. Therefore it can be considered to be against the best interests of the profession and, in the long term, against the public's interest.

The optometrist should never be influenced by any monetary or other financial factors while carrying out his professional duties. The unreasonably short time limits placed upon some practitioners are completely at odds with this ideal and are therefore deprecated.

Chapter 3
Patient Reception

3.1   Greeting, seating, and care of person and belongings

Patients attend a particular practice for a number of reasons; location, reputation, recommendation, cost, appearance, and also the helpfulness of the reception staff. The quality of magazines in the reception area, and the comfort of the seating are perhaps not decisive factors in a patient's choice of practice, but they can certainly affect the patient's perception of it. It is important to have sufficient comfortable (and suitable) seating for the usual number and variety of patients with which the practice deals. If the magazines are old and tatty then that may be the way in which the patient perceives the practice.

The receptionist is usually the first and last person with whom the patient deals and consequently can dramatically influence the success of the practice. It is therefore important to make sure that the reception staff are aware of this and behave in a helpful and courteous manner. This includes such aspects as making sure that the patient is comfortable, with space for their belongings in the reception or waiting area. Whenever possible the patient should be greeted by name. This may be difficult in a busy practice, or when a new receptionist is appointed, but at the very least, the receptionists should have details of all patients who are expected to attend the practice that day, so that they know which practitioner is examining which patient.

Patients should be encouraged to keep belongings with them so as to avoid any possibility of loss which could result in the practice (or one of the staff) being held liable. (There should be room in the consulting room for coats, hats and luggage which patients may bring with them.)

Answering the telephone is an important skill. Receptionists should be encouraged to do so quickly, and with a pleasant manner. It will not help the practice's reputation if, following ringing for five minutes, the telephone is answered by a harsh voice which simply says: ''ello'. It is worth having a standard answering phrase which the receptionists are encouraged to use, for example: 'Good morning (afternoon), I. Seemore Optometrists, how can I help you?'

The receptionists should always be aware of a practitioner's time keeping, and if a patient is likely to be delayed due to the optometrist's running late, then the patient should be advised accordingly. This should be couched in terms such as: 'I'm afraid Mr Seemore has been delayed slightly because he has had to deal with a patient with a very complicated problem. He should be with you in about. . . minutes. He will not rush your examination, just because he is running late, he devotes the same quality of care to all his patients.'

In some cases, a notice to this effect can usefully be displayed at the reception area.

3.2   The record card

When a patient has previously attended a particular practice, there should be a record card available. It is good practice to have the card available before the patient arrives, so that the reception staff can check such details as marital status, title, address, telephone number, and occupation, when the patient arrives.

There are a multitude of different types of record card, ranging from a simple blank sheet of paper to the most complex of designs which have a box or area for each and every possible test to which the patient could be subjected. The choice of card depends upon the practitioner, but can be influenced by external factors, such as storage area available, and whether there is any computerization of records. In all events a record card should be simple to read, and should allow the optometrist easy access to any relevant information about the patient.

The author's preference is for a simple card, blank except for the boxes for the patient's name, address, date of birth, telephone number, occupation, and GP's name. Continuation cards are blank except for a line at the top for the patient's name. This approach allows different practitioners (partners and associates) to complete a record in their own style, using whatever tests are appropriate and preferred for a particular patient and situation without wasting space by leaving inappropriate boxes or areas of card blank. The disadvantages of this system are that different optometrists record things differently, and a newcomer to the practice has to learn several different styles of writing and recording before he or she is easily able to interpret a particular record card.

Examples of two different formats and types of record cards are shown in Fig. 3.1. The first card type is the author's own, and its advantages have already been mentioned. The second card is one of the 'box' designs. It can be seen that it has no space available for 'extra' test such as fields, tonometry, colour vision, etc., and a new card is needed at alternate eye examinations (the reverse being similar in style to the front, without the personal details, but having spaces to record repairs carried out). The disadvantage of using cards such as this is that a lot of space will be wasted, and the card will appear untidy if any information other than that which is allowed for is recorded.

Some practitioners favour an envelope record form into which appropriate documents, spectacle frames, completed spectacles, or contact lenses may be placed. The author uses transparent polythene envelopes to contain the record card and any additions while an appliance is being processed, but the cards are filed without being so contained, to reduce storage space needed. Any letters or other documents which are to be kept with the card are firmly attached to it before filing.

The information on a record card should be regarded as confidential, and should never be mentioned to, or discussed with, anyone other than the patient without the express consent (preferably in writing) of the patient. The only exceptions to this are when sending a report to the patient's general medical practitioner, or when ordered to reveal information by a court of law.

(When preparing case records for the BCO PQEs, the candidate should ensure that all details which might personally identify a patient are obliterated so as to maintain their confidentiality.)

All ancillary staff who have access to the record cards should be instructed on the need for secrecy concerning the contents of the cards, and the inadvisability of entering into discussion with the patient on the subject of what is written on the card.

The position regarding ownership of the information on the card has not been clarified in a court of law, but is usually understood to lie with the principal of the practice. However, it is unreasonable to abuse this ownership by refusing to give another practitioner information which may be essential to allow adequate aftercare of the patient.

Where information about patients is stored using any form of electrical or magnetic media (such as computer discs or tapes) it is essential that the same precautions are observed as for a normal record card. Registration under the Data Protection Act 1984 is a legal requirement when such a form of recording is used. Details of registration can be obtained from:

The Registrar,
The Office of Data Protection,
Springfield House,
Water Lane,
Wilmslow,
Cheshire SK9 5AX
Tel: 0625 535777

3.3   Waiting area environment

The waiting area has already been described, and it is important not to overlook the fact that patients can often spend a significant amount of time in this area of the practice. Perhaps it is unreasonable but it is nevertheless true, that patients

Mr.
Mrs.
Miss

Address

Phone - Home

Post Code   Work

Date of Birth   Doctor

Occupation

Fig 3.1a   This is the record card used by the author. The reverse side is blank.

Mr Mrs Miss	Surname	Forenames	Date	Retest
			D.O.B.	Doctor
Address			Telephone	
			Occupation	
Previous Prescription	**R**		Hobbies & Sports	
	L		Media & Fondi	
History and Notes				

Phorias

	V	Sphere	Cylinder	Axis	Prism	Base	VA	ADD	VA	O.C.	
R											**D.N.I.B**
L											Tint

Date	Order	Frame Style	Colour	Eye	DBL	Side	Agle	HW	H/P	Cost	Collect
											Reference 196/067

Notes

			Date	Retest
			Media & Fundi	

Phorias

	V	Sphere	Cylinder	Axis	Prism	Base	VA	ADD	VA	O.C.	
R											**D.N.I.B**
L											Tint

Date	Order	Frame Style	Colour	Eye	DBL	Side	Agle	HW	H/P	Cost	Collected

Date	Order	Repair	Cost	Collected

Fig 3.1b An example of a 'box' design of record card, showing front and reverse sides.

tend to perceive the practitioner as being an integral part of his or her environment. This means that a scruffy, unwelcoming waiting area will give many patients the impression that those are the characteristics of the practitioner. These impressions are formed before meeting the practitioner and therefore can colour all the patient's subsequent behaviour.

It is a salutory experience to ask a professional colleague from another area to pass comment on the waiting area, or even to sit in it yourself and read the available literature for a few minutes. A few three-year-old magazines and a dog-eared leaflet from the Department of Health on the nicotine contents of various cigarettes are not a sign of a comfortable and cared-for reception/waiting area.

The waiting area is potentially a very powerful public relations and publicity resource. It is possible to inform patients about a vast range of professional functions which the optometrist can offer, and thus encourage them to ask about various services of which they might otherwise be unaware. There are a variety of excellent leaflets available from the optometric professional bodies, and also from various manufacturers, which can be usefully displayed. Naturally, the leaflet display should be kept neat and tidy, and should be regularly refilled.

Fresh flowers, whether in a vase or on the original plant, make a waiting room look attractive, and can also help mask any unpleasant odours from unwashed patients. Such flowers should be well maintained, and if a member of the practice staff is unable to carry out this task, a local garden centre may offer a contract flower maintenance service.

The waiting area should be slightly separated from the entrance and reception area, so that patients who are awaiting their appointment are allowed a degree of privacy, and do not feel that they are 'on display'. This does not mean that the patients are to be incarcerated in a pokey little room with no easy contact with the reception staff. Where possible, the reception area should be of an open plan nature and design, so as to appear inviting rather than intimidating. The waiting area, leading off the reception area should be *slightly* more enclosed to allow the mentioned feeling of privacy.

An important piece of equipment within the waiting room is a mirror, hand-held, wall mounted, or preferably both. Patients often like to have the chance to check their appearance before entering the consulting room.

Some practices have music playing, but with the wide variety of musical tastes, it is unlikely that any music will please most of the patients most of the time. If music is to be played within the waiting area (or even within the consulting room) then the permission of the copyright holder should first be obtained. The author is personally against such environmental pollution.

A tropical aquarium can be relaxing for patients to look at while they are waiting to enter the consulting room. It is most important that the unit is kept scrupulously clean, both for the sake of its appearance, and for the wellbeing of the fish.

Chapter 4
Preliminary Examination

This section of the examination starts as soon as the patient is seated in the consulting room, although even the gait and manner of entry may give the astute optometrist clues as to the possible problems from which the patient may be suffering. This section does not involve any physical contact with the patient (apart from possibly shaking hands).

By initially having a time which allows the patient to settle down within the consulting room environment without being 'tested' in any way, the patient is allowed to relax and gain confidence in the optometrist before the physical and physiological examinations are started. A relaxed patient is much more likely to respond well to the eye examination than one who is tense and feels threatened because he or she has not had a chance to form any sort of relationship with the optometrist.

The preliminary examination includes (silent) assessment of the appearance of the patient, the taking of history and symptoms, checking details of general health, medications, the familial ocular and general history, and occupation and hobbies. This assumes that details of name and address, telephone number, occupation, date of birth, and GP's name have been recorded by an assistant prior to the patient's entry into the consulting room. It is particularly worthwhile having the receptionist verify the name of the patient's GP before the patient enters the consulting room, as such a question from the practitioner can frighten some patients, as they imagine all manner of sinister reasons for it.

Some optometrists also like to include the checking of the patient's own spectacle correction in this section, although the author prefers to leave this element until after the refraction has been completed so as to avoid being influenced by previous findings.

The seat for the patient should be comfortable, and at a height which enables the patient to be seated without having to struggle. The illumination on the patient's face should not be set at its highest intensity as soon as the patient is seated; a bright light is essential for the external eye examination, but can intimidate the patient when she first sits in the chair.

14

Privacy during the examination is essential, and both the visual and auditory aspects of this should be considered. A patient who has overheard someone else's examination while in the waiting area is unlikely to be prepared to share details which she considers confidential.

It is useful, and on some occasions essential, to have a female assistant within immediate calling distance of the consulting room, to avoid the likelihood of being charged with any impropriety. It is advisable to insist that staff enter a consulting room immediately on knocking on the door, i.e. without waiting for an answer, and from time to time staff should be reminded of this, and the reason for so doing. Where a patient is known to be, or suspected of being a trouble maker in this sense, the assistant should be instructed to enter the consulting room at odd intervals during the eye examination. Inappropriate body contact should be avoided, as it will inevitably lead to problems for the optometrist, and the practitioner should always beware of any physical contact with an area of the patient's body other than the head.

4.1   General appearance

The assessment of the general appearance of the patient starts as soon as the first contact with the practitioner is made. The patient's general demeanour can give useful information which can aid in the final diagnostic process. The way in which a patient walks and talks can indicate many different types of neuro-muscular anomalies, even before the eye examination proper has started.

The patient's facial expression can often guide the astute clinician to select suitably worded questions and comments during the eye examination. Four typical facial groups are shown in Fig. 4.1.

Although features such as clothing and hairstyle may not be clinically relevant, they can indicate to the optometrist various features, and also give a rough guide as to the patient's possible interest in 'high tech' dispensing.

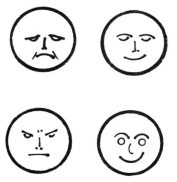

Fig. 4.1   Some facial types. First impressions may mislead but a patient's facial expression is usually some guide as to the approach required.

Patients may appear to be typical of various groups; the overweight and slightly sweaty person may be hypertensive; the thin and very 'twitchy' person may have an overactive thyroid. Of course, these features should only be regarded as of secondary importance when assessing the patient's eyes, but they can sometimes help confirm a tentative diagnosis.

The general appearance of the patient can be noted mentally and stored until it is linked with any other relevant factor. It is rarely a good idea to comment upon any particular feature to the patient unless it is of particular importance in determining the final diagnosis. Care should also be taken when recording such features on the record card; the laws of libel apply to patients' record cards!

Case study

Miss S.C., aged 19, was referred to me by the local hospital eye department for assessment of suitability for contact lens wear. As she entered the consulting room, I noticed that she had a slight stoop, and was quite tall. (In fact her height was 5ft 10in). As she sat down and reached for her handbag, I noticed that her fingers were quite long, and then also that her limbs were slightly longer than usual. She presented me with a referral letter from the hospital optometrist which stated that she was 'very myopic with bilateral dislocation of lenses'. On slit lamp microscopy, I found that the crystalline lenses were both displaced upwards and slightly temporally, and made a tentative diagnosis of Marfan's syndrome. She admitted having an 'odd shaped chest bone' (pectus excavatum), and a highly arched palate. The diagnosis was confirmed by the referring eye department staff. The rest of this patient's record is unremarkable for this section of the text, but she is now wearing hard gas-permeable contact lenses, and can see well enough to have passed her driving test. Her son (born 1987) shows no sign of the condition. A photograph of this patient's hand is shown in Fig. 4.2.

4.2   Occupation, sports, hobbies and driving

When a record card already exists for a patient, some of these details may already be recorded. They can help in the choice of suitable comments with which to make the patient realize that the optometrist is interested in the patient as an individual. However, it is always worthwhile asking the patient whether she is still doing the same job, has any new hobbies, or has started (or ceased) driving a motor vehicle.

When descriptions of employment such as 'self employed', 'sales executive', 'local government employee', or 'engineer' are given, it is important that the optometrist finds out exactly what type of working environment the patient is in. A 'self employed' person can be anything from a senior partner in a firm of management consultants to someone who works in his or her own fish and chip van. Local government employees range from road cleaners to the town clerk. Sales executives can range from someone working behind the counter in the local hardware shop to an international 'jet-setting' representative for a computer company. The term 'engineer' is likewise frequently mis-used by mechanics and technicians, from those involved in the repair of crashed cars to those making the internal workings for computers. The eliciting of exact occupation and therefore visual requirements should be done tactfully; some patients can be very self-aware and slightly embarrassed when revealing their jobs. The author suffered a degree of embarrassment when, on asking a young lady who had given her occupation as 'public relations and entertainment' exactly what sort of work she did, received the explanation: 'Well, actually, I'm a stripper. . .'.

Patients who hold a driving licence, or a pilot's licence should have the fact noted and the practitioner should make sure that they are aware of the appropriate visual requirements for the type of licence, ensuring that the patient is able to fulfill them. If, at the end of the eye examination, it appears that the requirements cannot be met by the patient, suitable advice should be given, and the fact noted on the record card. Sometimes it may be advisable to give such patients a written statement which records their visual performance, and the advice given. A copy of the statement should always be kept and attached to the patient's record card.

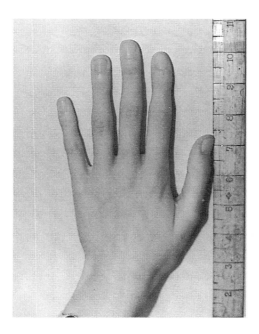

Fig. 4.2 Marfan's syndrome. Hand features are characteristic.

Case study

Mr P.C., a solicitor aged 48, consulted an optometrist for a routine eye examination, wishing to be fitted with contact lenses. He had just taken up playing squash and found that his executive bifocal spectacles were not as suitable on the court as 'in court'. He was markedly myopic, (circa – 8.00 in both eyes) and his father had suffered from a retinal detachment. The optometrist suggested that he be fitted with a pair of spectacles suitably designed to afford adequate protection to the eyes from the squash ball (and racket). He accepted the recommendation and a Marwitz 7010 frame glazed with polycarbonate lenses was dispensed. He subsequently returned to thank the optometrist for his advice, as a ball had hit one of the lenses of his spectacles 'straight off the opponent's racket', but happily he had not been injured. Had he been wearing contact lenses, he could have easily suffered a serious injury.

4.3   Symptoms

This area of the eye examination leads nicely on from the history-taking. It is important to note, where possible, the patient's own description of the presenting symptoms, although occasionally the patient may be excessively verbose and a contracted form may be desirable in order to save space on the record card.

Symptoms can be divided into a number of categories, depending on the approach of the individual optometrist. The essentials of symptom recording, however, are details of the type, location, severity, onset and duration, association, and period suffered.

When recorded logically, the symptoms can often guide the practitioner towards likely causes even before the physical eye examination has commenced.

Recording symptoms

Symptom recording can be by various abbreviations to suit the taste, requirements and record card space of the practitioner. Typical examples are presented below, followed by their 'interpretation'.

Notes on record

　　　　c/o fr. h/a after 2hrs. n/v past 6/12.

Expanded, this means:
Patient complains of frontal headaches after two hours of near vision, over the past six months.

Table 4.1

Abbreviation	Translates as
?/365	? days
?/52	? weeks
?/12	? months
d/v	distance vision
n/v	near vision
hor	horizontal
ver	vertical
c/o	complains of
fr	frontal
temp	temporal
h/a	headaches
asth	asthenopia
dip	diplopia

Notes on record

c/o asth. post V.D.U. & hor.dip. D/V a.m. 3/52

Expanded, this means:
Patient complains of eye ache and discomfort after using a visual display unit, and horizontal diplopia in the mornings, over the past three weeks.

Descriptions of symptoms

Sometimes patients may give the most peculiar descriptions of their symptoms, such as 'wriggling eyeballs', 'zoomy vision', or 'blotches'. Such means of describing symptoms may be completely accurate and meaningful to the patient, but obviously require some further investigation so as to elucidate the precise nature of the problem.

One of the most important areas of symptom-taking is the accurate recording of the time factors; onset, frequency, and duration. These aspects can be vital when deciding upon the eventual diagnosis and action to be taken. For example, a patient complaining of diplopia for the past few days will be assessed in a different light to one who has suffered from similar symptoms for the past twenty years. Likewise a patient complaining of 'flashes of light' since being hit in the eye the previous week will be assessed differently to someone presenting with similar symptoms but having experienced them for the previous fifteen years.

There are several abbreviations which are frequently used when recording symptoms, as the above examples have demonstrated. A few of the more commonly used ones are presented in Table 4.1. (This list is not meant to be exhaustive, and each practitioner will, of course, have some personal favourites which are particularly appropriate to his or her own style and practice.)

There are some abbreviations which are occasionally used to describe the mental or personality categories into which a patient may fall. These are usually libellous, and their use is strongly discouraged.

To some extent the actual wording of a question to a patient can determine the answer; the optometrist should be careful in the selection of questions, and should not ask leading questions unless a particular situation necessitates them. For example, if a patient complains of headaches, the duration, location and association need to be established. This should be done using neutral questioning, such as: 'when do you get the headaches?' If a question such as: 'Do you get the headaches when you read a lot?' is posed, then the patient may give the answer that she believes the optometrist expects or wants, rather than give a 'wrong' answer. When inaccurately used, the leading form of question can actually obscure important information, as the replies to such questions are frequently monosyllabic, and the patient may thus feel that expansion on the answers given is not wanted.

Asthenopia, or ocular discomfort, can be caused by many factors. Among the more common are:
1   Uncorrected refractive errors, particularly those which cause accommodative stress;
2   Uncompensated heterophorias;
3   Poor (inadequate, excessive or badly positioned) lighting.
Most forms of asthenopia are caused by one or more of these factors, and it is usually well within the professional abilities of an optometrist to suggest a 'cure'. One of the common, but frequently neglected, symptoms is that of pressure or discomfort behind the eyes. This is often due to the patient 'screwing up his eyes' for prolonged periods. This action, anatomically the prolonged contraction of the orbicularis oculi muscles, can cause pressure upon the globe, and hence push it backwards, thus causing symptoms of retro-bulbar pressure or discomfort. The ciliary muscle and accessory muscles of accommodation can also cause pain referred to the retrobulbar region when over-used. The symptoms are usually cured by allowing the patient the means to see without having to 'screw up his eyes', or by relieving the accommodative stress.

Photophobia can be defined as abnormal sensitivity to light which causes the patient discomfort or difficulty when performing particular visual tasks. There are many different causes of photophobia, ranging from corneal opacities at one end of the eye, to poorly functioning retinal pigment epithelium at the other. When the patient has had the symptoms recorded, a careful eye examination will usually reveal the cause of the problem, and a means of alleviating it. This may involve advice on lighting, tinted spectacle lenses, or occasionally referral for medical attention.

(It has been suggested that some patients develop 'psychological' photophobia, and wear tinted lenses in a sub-conscious attempt to hide themselves from the outside world. The author has heard this theory being proposed by an optometrist who specialized in hypnosis, but has never come across the problem himself.)

4.4 History

An existing record card may give some degree of background; it is, however, always worthwhile checking the facts, and altering them if necessary.

When the patient has not been examined previously at the practice a full history should be taken. This should include details of the patient's previous correction(s), and any ocular surgery, trauma, or therapy.

The patient may be eager to discuss some interesting background facts, but should not be allowed to ramble on with irrelevant descriptions of what treatment had been prescribed by the village herbalist for a grandmother's sticky eyes, or why he has had ringing in his ears ever since an operation for ingrowing toenails.

The art in history-taking is initially to ask questions which should have short (ideally single word) answers. Once basic information has been gleaned from the patient, more leading questions which invite slightly longer answers can be asked should there be any unclear details. Where possible, dates should be noted, as they can sometimes have a bearing on subsequent advice to the patient. A 'case example' is included here as a guide, although the details will naturally vary with each patient.

Notes on record

> Last ex. 2 yrs. by I. Seemore. = N/V Rx. N/V Rx.15 yrs. No D/V Rx. Iritis L.E. 1966, treated with Oc, nil since.

Expanded, this means:

Last eye examination two years ago carried out by an optometrist called I. Seemore, resulting in the dispensing of a new near vision prescription. (Note: if dispensed elsewhere this should be noted.) Patient has worn correction for close work for the past 15 years, but has never had a distance correction. Patient suffered from Iritis in the left eye in 1966; this was treated with eyedrops, and there has been no recurrence since then.

The history will often give clues as to possible problems. For example, a patient may comment about a retinal detachment treated a few years ago (this sort of comment should always prompt the optometrist to enquire about any family history of the mentioned condition); the optometrist will be on the look-out for vitreous floaters, possible myopia, and any sign of retinal disease or degeneration which may be connected with the earlier detachment. Hopefully, at the conclusion of the eye examination, the optometrist will advise the patient about care of the eyes; avoiding contact sports such as boxing and comments about the need to seek urgent attention should any of the usual symptoms of retinal detachment occur.

Some patients may have spent time abroad. This should be recorded, and the patient should be asked about any particular drugs taken while in foreign parts, for example, anti-malarials. Tropical climates, and also the increased levels of visible and invisible radiation can all affect the visual system. The optometrist should subsequently be on the look-out for any sign of active or past disease which may have a connection with the time spent abroad, and the side-effects of any drugs used.

4.5   General health and medications

It is important that the patient be asked whether any drugs or other medications are being taken or otherwise used, and a note made of the reply. Many drugs have ocular or visual side-effects, and if the practitioner has no knowledge of the patient's medications, it is possible to arrive at an incorrect diagnosis.

The consulting room library should include a current edition of *MIMS* as well as the common books on ocular pharmacology.

When recording a patient's medications, the drug name and dosage, the duration of the treatment, and the reason for the treatment should be noted. Some patients may carry details of their medications with them, but if the patient is unable to remember the name of the drug being taken, they should be requested to contact the optometrist with the appropriate details as soon as convenient, should an adverse reaction be suspected. On the author's practice appointment cards there is the subscript:

> 'Please bring details of any medications when you come for your eye examination.'

This often proves to be a helpful reminder to those patients with poor memory for drug names, and can save a lot of time when completing the record card.

4.6   Family general and ocular history

Following the questions about the patient's own general health, medications, and history, the patient should be asked about any relevant familial conditions. Many optometric conditions are familial, so it is important to be aware of such potential problems before the eye examination proper is started.

A few questions along the lines of:

'Has anyone in the family ever had cataracts or glaucoma?'

'Do you have any relatives with problems with their eyes?'

'Are there any members of your family with chronic health problems?'

will usually produce sufficient relevant information. If the replies are vague, seek clarification. In the interests of time management, it may be necessary to 'encourage' the patient to get to the point. This should be done tactfully as patients are often delighted to have what they see as a chance to relate their family saga.

Mini quiz on inherited conditions
Which of the following conditions are likely to be inherited?

1 Glaucoma	7 Coloboma
2 Albinism	8 Deutranopia
3 Aphakia	9 Persistent pupillary membrane
4 Keratoconus	10 Microphthalmia
5 Nystagmus	11 Retinitis pigmentosa
6 Follicular conjunctivitis	12 Chalazion

Answer: All except 3, 6, 9 and 12.

Case study

Miss S.P, aged 13, was brought for an eye examination as she had been seen rubbing her eyes frequently over the previous few weeks. She had no visual complaints, and had never previously consulted anyone about her eyes. She was in good health, and was not taking any medication. The refractive and oculomotor examinations were unremarkable, and she had excellent acuities, good accommodation, and ophthalmoscopy showed no abnormalities of the internal eye. However, the external eye examination showed mild conjunctival hyperaemia, and on everting the lids, small papillae were found on both upper tarsal conjunctivae. Although the mother had initially said that there was no family history of any general health problems, on re-questioning, she mentioned that the patient's younger sister suffered from eczema, and that her father had allergic rhinitis. Having completed the examination, the patient was referred to her general medical practitioner for investigation of allergic conjunctivitis. It transpired that the young lady had recently been given a hamster, and was in the habit of allowing it to sit on her hand and 'kiss' her face. Much to the young lady's dismay the doctor suggested removing the hamster. This was done, the ocular reaction was resolved, and the eye rubbing ceased.

4.7   Current spectacles

The checking of the patient's existing spectacles is essential before any decisions are taken concerning the prescribing of a new correction. All spectacles which the patient actually uses should be checked. The following details should be noted:

- Dioptric power
- Optical centration distance (distance and near)
- Lens material, and form

- Bifocal/multifocal/varifocal type
- Reading addition
- Tints or coatings
- Scratches or other flaws
- Physical condition of frame, including details of breaks, cracks, or corrosion.

Sometimes it becomes obvious that advice on the handling or cleaning of spectacles needs to be given; this should be done tactfully. Where appropriate a demonstration can be given. Inspecting the spectacle case is often a good idea, giving insight into the standard of care given by the patient.

The patient's own spectacles should be handled carefully and kept in a safe place during the examination, or returned to the patient as soon as convenient.

Chapter 5
External Examination

This part of the routine eye examination follows the preliminary section. It involves some physical contact with the patient's face, but hopefully the patient will be sufficiently at ease to allow this to proceed without problem. All of this section can be completed without extinguishing all the lights and this allows the patient a further period to settle before everything goes dark.

The individual elements of this part can and should be arranged so that they flow easily. For example, the inspection of the lids, lashes, conjunctiva, cornea, anterior chamber, and pupillary reactions may all be done together, as they involve use of the hand slit-lamp. Likewise, the assessment of ocular motility, convergence, and visual fields can be carried out as a group, using the same target. (The author uses a 3 mm diameter white map-pin mounted on a six-inch black pencil as a target for these tests.)

It is often useful, and always reassuring to the patient, to make some brief comment as to what is being done and what the particular test or technique is expected to show.

Hygiene is an essential part of professional optometry, and this is most important during the physical examination of the external eyes, when the ocular region of the face is touched by the practitioner. The optometrist should always wash his hands immediately before commencing the actual examination procedure.

Bodily odours, tainted breath, and strong perfumes are all hazardous for good relationships between optometrists and patient. Optometrists who enjoy curry or other spicy foods should avoid eating them when they are likely to be examining patients on the following day. Where this is unavoidable, mouth fresheners such as Amplex or Listerine are advisable.

5.1   Unaided vision

This should be tested using British Standard Snellen charts for distance, and one of the recognized near test types, such as that recommended by the Faculty of Ophthalmologists. The testing should be done under appropriate illumination, and each eye tested individually.

Where possible the weaker eye should be tested first so that there is no possibility of the patient 'cheating' by remembering the letters. It is also a good idea to ask the patient to read out the smallest letters he or she can see, rather than getting them to read out the whole chart.

Children may have to be assisted by using a letter or symbol matching test; this can often be done as a 'game'. When testing children (and sometimes this is true for adults) the object used to occlude the non-tested eye should be held in place by the practitioner to avoid pressure being applied to the globe and causing corneal deformation and resulting in a temporary blurring of vision. Some children may object to having something held in front of their eye; it is advisable for the optometrist to demonstrate the correct positioning of the occluder before allowing the individual to take over the task.

Some practitioners prefer to record the unaided vision for each eye before any other section of the eye examination is carried out, so as to avoid the possibility of a patient later complaining that her eyes have deteriorated as a result of the eye examination procedures themselves.

5.2   Posture: general and head

The patient's general posture can indicate a great deal about health, background, and psyche. There are several books on the subject of 'body language' which give insight into this interesting field, although pathological posture problems, such as those caused by cervical spondylosis or scoliokyphosis are outside the scope of such texts.

Patients who habitually stand, sit or walk in an unusual manner may well have different visual requirements to a patient with 'normal' posture or gait. This should be carefully considered when making decisions about prescribing suitable spectacles. For example, the bifocal type and positioning may have to be adjusted to a different position from the 'normal' of level with the lower lid margins in a patient who habitually holds his or her head at an odd angle due to a neck or spine deformity. In such cases particular care should be given to determining the working environment and occupational visual demands which the patient has to meet.

An odd posture or head position can frequently indicate some form of oculomotor anomaly, so appropriate binocular vision tests should be carried out to determine the type of problem present.

5.3   Skin: texture and irregularities

The skin, which is one of the largest organs of the body, forms a protective, waterproof, elastic and sensitive covering.

The skin has several functions:

- Protection of the underlying structures from physical, chemical, or pathogenic assault.
- Acting as a sense organ for pain, temperature and touch.
- Temperature regulation.
- Excretion and consequent assistance in fluid and mineral metabolism.
- Vitamin D production by action of ultraviolet 'light'.
- Signalling information to others about the physical and mental state of the subject.

Several of these functions are relevant when considering the skin around the eyes. For example, acting as a sense organ for touch, the lid skin performs a primary protective function for the eyes, and can thereby prevent damage to the globe.

The facial skin is probably more exposed to the 'elements' and therefore consequent damage than any other area of skin, save perhaps that of the hands. It is also possibly more exposed to various cosmetic chemicals than any other single area of the body. These features can make the correct identification of skin irregularities difficult, and dermatology is obviously outside the scope of this book. (There are several good pocket texts on skin diseases available for the interested practitioner and one should be available in every practice library.)

Any irregularities of the skin around the eyes should be noted, and when verbal description is inadequate, diagrams should be used to demonstrate the location and size of the defect. The ideal way of recording skin defects and irregularities is a photograph, as this can allow accurate monitoring of any change in size, shape or colour. If colour rendering is important, a small range of colour samples should be included within the frame of the photograph. The patient may comment upon the skin irregularity and tell the practitioner how long it has been present. This can obviously help with decision making when referral to a physician is being contemplated. However, the patient's word should never be regarded as unerringly accurate as memory is frequently at odds with reality.

The usual skin irregularities found around the eyes can be divided into three categories:

1 Innocent, congenital marks, such as moles and other pigmentary blemishes.
2 Signs of systemic or localized disease, such as the thickening which is associated with eczema, or the erythema associated with acne rosacea.
3 Signs of skin reaction to insult, such as scars, and areas of differing skin texture due to pressure from spectacle frames.

These categories are by no means separate, and can frequently coexist.

The skin anomalies most commonly encountered in general optometric practice are eczema, dermatitis of various types, and basal cell carcinomas. The last of these deserves special mention due to its increasing frequency, partly due to the increasing average age of the British population, and partly due to more exposure to ultraviolet radiation. If a basal cell carcinoma is suspected, the patient should be referred to their GP after the optometrist has measured and sketched, or photographed the lesion. Although such tumours are generally of the slow-growing variety, early excision is usually advised.

The assessment of the facial and particularly the peri-ocular skin can often be carried out silently while talking to the patient during the preliminary sections of the examination, such as history and symptoms. However, some leisons may not be noticed until the patient's spectacles have been removed, or until the optometrist looks carefully at the patient's face, as spectacles can sometimes abuse or displace the nasal canthus and associated structures.

5.4   Lids and lashes

The examination of the eyes, as understood by many patients, begins with the inspection of the lids and eyelashes. As mentioned in the introduction, it is important that the practitioner washes his or her hands before touching the patient's face, and is seen (or at least heard) doing so.

The lashes are the last line of defence which the eyes have against the debris in the atmosphere, and are therefore important in the maintenance of ocular health. Positioning of potentially toxic or irritative substances inside the eyelash margin should be discouraged.

The lids and lashes should first be observed with the eyes in the primary position noting any obvious irregularities of structure or position. This may include ptosis, ectropion, entropion, scars, scanty or missing lashes, styes, and trichiasis.

It is important to maintain a light hand; gentle handling of the lids will help prevent or at least minimize any possibility of blepharospasm, reassuring the patient as to the optometrist's abilities in general. A patient is unlikely to trust a practitioner who cannot handle the lids with gentleness and ease. Gentle handling of the lids is also required when the patient is wearing any make-up; she will not thank you for smudging it.

Sometimes absence of lashes can be self-inflicted rather than due to alopecia or other skin disease. A case study to illustrate this follows.

Case study
Miss S.J.P., aged 10, was brought for an eye examination by her mother. The child had been seen rubbing her eyes frequently and vigorously, but denying any irritation. There were no visual symptoms. The external examination of the eyes showed nearly total absence of the lashes from both sets of lids. There was no history of skin or hair disorder, and no erythema or other abnormal skin features were visible. There was no significant refractive error, and the vision, oculomotor balance, colour vision and ophthalmoscopy were all within normal limits. Slit-lamp examination showed healthy lids and palpebral and bulbar conjunctivae.

There were some fine lashes present on both set of lids, but most of the follicles had stumps of lashes present which were just level with the skin surface. On inspection under higher magnification the ends of the lash stumps appeared to be almost square-ended. The child was asked if she ever plucked at her lashes, and she admitted doing so when at school. She was advised to cease, and a further examination was advised three months later.

When she attended for the follow-up examination there was little change in the state of the lashes. The child was asked to leave the consulting room, and her mother was questioned on possible sources of stress. It was revealed that the family was under a lot of tension as the father had left the home suddenly, and also the child was being bullied at school. A discussion with the form teacher was recommended and TLC (tender loving care) advised. The child was examined again three months later, when the eyelashes were found to have regrown. The mother commented that the teacher had not been aware of the home situation or the bullying, and having been made aware, had managed to help the child overcome some of her difficulties.

5.5   Conjunctiva

The examination of the conjunctiva follows naturally from the inspection of the lids and lashes.

The lids should be *gently* lifted away from the globes. The insides of both upper and lower lids, along with the surface of the globe are inspected. The patient is asked to look upwards when inspecting the lower areas of conjunctiva, and vice versa. The lacrimal gland is often not visible when looking under the upper lids. Obvious visibility of one or both lacrimal glands may indicate either a localized or systemic problem, and the patient should be referred.

The medial and lateral canthi should also be checked. To allow easy inspection, the patient should be asked to look to the left and right. Patients showing confusion as to left and right can be assisted by a tactful tap on the appropriate shoulder.

When examining the inner canthi, particular attention should be paid to the lacrimal puncta. Their size and position should be noted if abnormal. If the patient has complained of watering eyes, or any other symptoms which might indicate poor tear drainage, then the patency of the puncta should be tested. This is best done using sodium fluorescein solution instilled into the lower conjunctival sac. Gentle (digital) pressure on the lids at the position of the canaliculi should normally cause some regurgitation of the tear fluid, and when fluorescein is used in conjunction with a Burton lamp, the patency is easily demonstrated. Full patency of the naso-lacrimal ducts can also be checked using this method, although blowing of the nose (on to a tissue rather than a fabric handkerchief) by the patient is necessary in order to check if any fluorescein-containing tear fluid has passed through the ducts. Occasionally it is necessary to check the back of the patient's throat (visually) using a Burton lamp, as some patients tend to drain tear fluid backwards through the nose rather than forwards.

There are many ways of illuminating and observing the conjunctiva: focal illumination using a hand slit lamp and loupe; the ophthalmoscope; the major slit-lamp microscope; naked eye and diffuse illumination. These techniques are well described in other texts. However, a word of warning for the potential BCO PQE candidate: please make sure that you have mastered whichever technique you use during the examination. Poorly practised and inexpert use of a method is very obvious to the examiners, and will not do anything to impress them.

When any abnormality of the palpebral or bulbar conjunctiva is detected, the lid should be fully everted to allow complete inspection (Figs. 5.1 and 5.2). This procedure should also be carried out when there is any history or symptoms of an allergic ocular reaction.

Everting the upper lids takes practice, but is a technique well worth acquiring, as many oddities can lurk unsuspected underneath. The easiest method is gently but firmly to grasp the margin and lashes of the upper lid with the right hand as near to the lid as possible, and then to pull the lid slightly down and away from the globe. The tip of the left index finger may then be used to push the tarsal plate

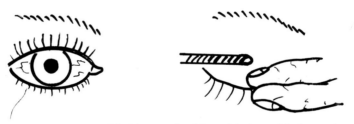

Fig. 5.1 Eversion of the upper eyelid. Observe the lids and lashes with the eye open. Direct patient to look down. Place fulcrum at upper edge of tarsal plate. Grasp edge of upper lid. Remind patient to look down.

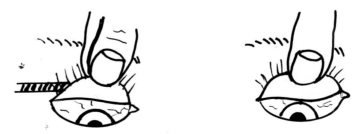

Fig. 5.2 Upper lid everted. Finger and thumb have lifted lid, bringing it forward and up to fold over the fulcrum. One digit holds lid and patient still looks down, after fulcrum is removed.

down while lifting the lid margin upwards, thus flipping the lid over. If the optometrist has large fingers, or is nervous or clumsy, then the use of a plastic rod, or even a pen, may be helpful. It is best to perfect the technique with the co-operation of a friend or relative before trying it out on an unsuspecting patient!

It is quite difficult strictly to define 'normal' for the palpebral (or bulbar) conjunctiva except in a negative way. Thus normal appearance can be regarded as the absence of any abnormalities such as vascular congestion and dilatation, cysts, concretions, follicles, papillae, foreign bodies or other lesions (see Figs. 5.3–5.6).

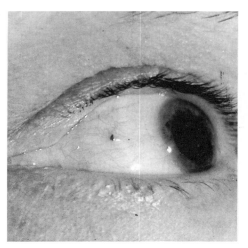

Fig. 5.3 Conjunctival foreign body.

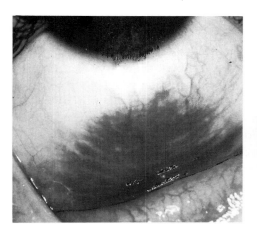

Fig. 5.5 Subconjunctival ecchymosis. Following some head trauma such sub-conjunctival haemorrhage could suggest a skull fracture.

Fig. 5.4 Injected vessels on bulbar conjunctive. Note arcus just within the limbus.

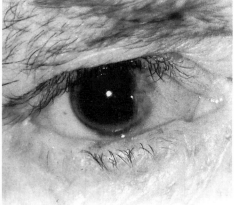

Fig. 5.6 Corneal infiltration. The nasal cornea has suffered encroachment of opaque tissue.

Foreign bodies can frequently lodge under the upper lids, and become partially embedded in the palpebral conjunctiva unless removed without undue delay. The most common area for these to lodge is within the central lid area, between 4 and 10 mm from the lid margin. They can sometimes be detected by the tell-tale tracks which they leave on the corneal epithelium which stains well with sodium fluorescein. If the foreign body is superficial (and the assessment of this is always a situation in which the use of a slit-lamp microscope is mandatory), then it may be gently lifted off the conjunctival surface using a fresh clean (sterile if possible) cotton bud, or freshly disinfected loop of nylon line (fine fishing line is ideal).

Any abnormalities of structure or appearance should be noted and where appropriate, a diagram is drawn.

The conjunctiva is classified as a mucous membrane, and therefore should exhibit that feature which is common to such structures throughout the body — it should be WET. It is usually wetted by the tears, although contact lens solutions, eye irrigation lotions, and topical ocular medications can all 'wet' it. This brings the topic of tears to our consideration. The tear film should be assessed by noting the regularity and 'sheen' of the cornea. The tear film reservoir at the lid margins and at the inner canthi can also be observed, and if a more accurate note of tear function is indicated (due to symptoms or signs which could indicate poor quality or quantity of tear fluid) then there are several techniques which can be used. The most frequently used of these techniques are:

1   Tear volume assessment – using a Schirmer strip.
2   Tear break-up time – using sodium fluorescein.
3   Tear production – assessed by dilution of a suitable dye, such as sodium fluorescein.
4   Tear film durability – assessed by observing the stability of keratometer mires. Tear film break-up time assessment can often give useful guidance to the alert practitioner regarding the particular cause of the problems. A patient with poor quality or deficient mucus production (due to inactive or absent conjunctival goblet cells) will usually show a consistent pattern of tear film break-up; the tear film will frequently break up in the same place. This type of appearance can also be caused by corneal epithelial scars, so careful slit-lamp microscopy should always be carried out. Irregularities in the location of the tear film break-up can be caused by either the aqueous or lipid layers being of poor quality or quantity.

Where any invasive technique is used, the patient should be fully informed about the procedure, and consent obtained PRIOR to starting. Any drugs or other agents used on the eye should be noted.

5.6   Cornea and anterior chamber

Examination of the cornea and anterior chamber requires focal illumination, usually provided by a pen torch or hand slit-lamp. Unless a major slit-lamp microscope is immediately available, the practitioner should also use a loupe to allow fine structures to be more easily seen.

The slit beam should initially be focused on the lateral limbus, then gradually moved across the cornea, while the optometrist watches for any irregularities in the structure of the cornea. It is possible to use several of the lighting techniques used during major slit-lamp microscopy with a hand slit-lamp and loupe, such as scleral scatter, direct, and diffuse illumination.

Whenever a patient has any conjunctival injection, or complains of soreness or foreign body sensation, sodium fluorescein solution (either from a freshly opened 'Minim' or a freshly opened and saline impregnated 'Fluorette') should be used in conjunction with a Burton lamp or a major slit-lamp microscope to check corneal integrity.

Corneal sensitivity can be measured using an anaesthesiometer, but such instruments are uncommon in general optometric practice. If sensitivity assessment is indicated, a wisp of fresh cotton wool can be used to stimulate a blink reflex and thus estimate gross sensitivity. The wisp of cotton wool should be brought towards the patient's eye from the temporal side so as to avoid the patient seeing it and provoking an unwanted blink reflex (Fig. 5.7).

The depth of the anterior chamber can be estimated, although it is advisable to limit the estimate to four gradings; deep, average, shallow, and dangerously shallow. The central anterior chamber depth does not always give an indication of the 'angle', and it is therefore advisable to estimate the anterior chamber angle as close to the limbus as possible, as well as the anterior chamber depth. Van Herrick's grading can be used for this (Fig. 5.8).

The keratometer, or a placido disc (more commonly in the form of a Klein keratoscope) can be used to assist location and diagnosis of any corneal irregularities or foreign bodies. The tear film quality can also be partially judged with these methods. The author has seen (and used) a home-made version of a placido disc, constructed from a white hemispherical plastics vegetable strainer which had a + 5.00 lens placed at its vertex. External illumination was required, but the 'instrument' was easy to use, gave a good image, and was very cheap! (See Fig. 5.9.)

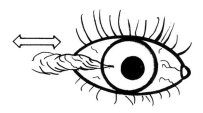

Fig. 5.7 Test for corneal sensitivity. A wisp of cotton wool is advanced from the temporal side of the cornea, avoiding the cilia and without undue visual warning to the patient.

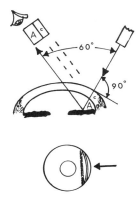

Fig. 5.8 Van Herrick grading. Anterior chamber depth relative to corneal thickness is assessed close to the limbus.

It is possible to detect many defects of pupillary structure using the hand slit-lamp; indeed, some dangerous lesions, such as malignant melanomas of the ciliary body causing the iris to bulge forwards slightly into the anterior chamber may go undetected unless the optometrist uses some form of slit-lamp, either hand-held or a major version. On several occasions the author has detected a suspicious bulge in a patient's iris using a hand slit-lamp. All these patients were referred for ophthalmological assessment, and one proved to have a melanoma of the iris root. (The rest had simple iris cysts.)

Case Study

Miss J.L., aged 29, had been under my care as a contact lens patient for several years with no signs or symptoms. At one of her routine annual check-up appointments, I noticed a small bulge in the periphery of the right iris at 3 o/c. This was only apparent using the slit-lamp microscope, when the gap between the iris and the back surface of the cornea was considerably narrowed in one area. There was no sign of change or irregularity of the surrounding iris pigment, and the refraction was stable, with no alteration in astigmatism. The patient was referred to her general medical practitioner, who, not having a slit-lamp microscope, referred her to an ophthalmologist. The lesion was diagnosed as an innocent iris cyst (after three appointments) and she was discharged back to my care.

Some surgical procedures, such as cataract extraction, naturally affect the iris, and these changes should be recorded. Diagrams are useful when recording any defects of structure within the anterior portion of the globe, and should be clear, of a reasonable size, and labelled where necessary.

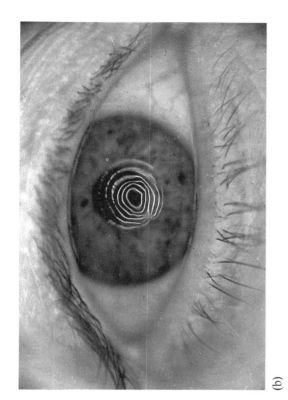

(b)

Fig. 5.9 Placido disc reflections. (a) Cornea is relatively normal centrally, with mid-peripheral distortion of the images. Does the oval shape of the more central rings suggest slight 'against the rule' toricity of the cornea? (b) Keratoconus, with patient fixating centrally. (c) The same keratoconus patient, now fixating slightly to the temporal side. Note the reflections from the sclera. (Photographs by the late E. F. Fincham)

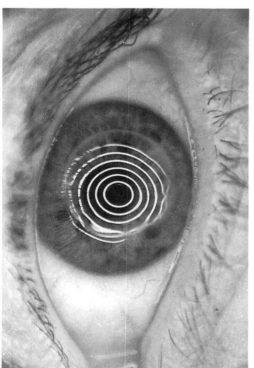

(a)

(c)

If there is anything unusual about the colour of the irides, or the texture or arrangement of the fibres, it should be noted. Any particular differences of pigmentation, either between the eyes, or on one eye, should be noted, and where appropriate, a diagram drawn. The practitioner should be alert to the possibility of a patient suffering from Horner's syndrome whenever heterochromia irides is present. Horner's syndrome is caused by a partial or total interruption of the sympathetic nerve supply anywhere along its route from the hypothalamus to the eye, and is characterized by the following features:

1   Slight ptosis due to paralysis of Muller's muscle.
2   Slight elevation of the lower lid due to paralysis of the smooth muscle linked to the lower tarsal plate.
3   Apparent enophthalmos due to the narrowing of the vertical palpebral aperture caused by (1) and (2).
4   Miosis, which is more apparent in low levels of illumination. (The pupillary reactions to light and near stimuli are not affected.)
5   Reduced perspiration on the affected side of the face if the causative lesion is below the superior cervical ganglion.
6   Slightly increased accommodation, due to unopposed action of the parasympathetic nerve supply.
7   Heterochromia irides, more usually present if the condition is congenital or has been acquired during infancy.

Unusually dark or light areas of iris should alert the optometrist to the possibility of abnormal (active) pigment production or destruction. The possible causes of such features are many and varied, and a patient exhibiting any such irregularity should be referred to their general medical practitioner for further investigation. The optometrists should always make a complete record of his own findings for possible future reference. Again, diagrams, or better still, photographs, are advisable.

Persistent pupillary membranes are quite common, and can be observed using an ophthalmoscope or with a slit-lamp microscope. Although they are of no significance unless they restrict the movement of the iris, an element of professional satisfaction can be gained from noting them, and the 'completeness' of the patient's record is enhanced (see Fig. 5.10).

5.7   Pupillary reactions

Following on from the above, with the pen torch still in the optometrist's hand, the pupil reactions should be checked.

Three main pupillary reactions (direct, consensual, and near) should be stimulated, because they each use different pathways, and differential diagnosis of various neurological lesions can thus be aided. The direct and consensual reflexes can be checked using the pen torch, or hand slit-lamp. Some practitioners prefer

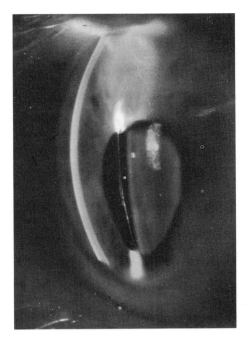

Fig. 5.10 Persistent pupillary membrane. The patient also had a congenital coloboma and this slit–lamp section shows an unusually displaced pupil. (Photo by the late E. F. Fincham)

to use the ophthalmoscope, but the author feels that this is rather like using a binocular microscope to inspect postage stamps; possible, but a little unwieldy! The near reflex can be tested by asking the patient to look into the distance, perhaps towards the consulting room mirror, or at the test chart, and then to look at a small target held about 10 to 15 cm in front of the patient's face.

During ophthalmoscopy, while looking into one eye with the ophthalmoscope it is difficult to observe the other pupil's reaction. For this reason, as well as the ergonomic consideration of having the pen torch immediately to hand, this section has been placed here within the routine, rather than within the ophthalmoscopy section.

A defect in one reaction, while another is normal, can give some information about the location of the cause of the defect. For example, if the right pupil reacts fully to direct and near stimuli, but not to consensual stimulation, and the left pupil reacts to consensual and near stimuli, but not to direct stimulation, then the tentative diagnosis of absence of light perception in the left eye might be made. This can be confirmed by checking the vision. There are many different ways in which the pupils can react which can signify different problems. The reader is advised to find a clear diagram of the visual pathway showing the light reflex pathways. This will help immensely when trying to locate the cause of any but the

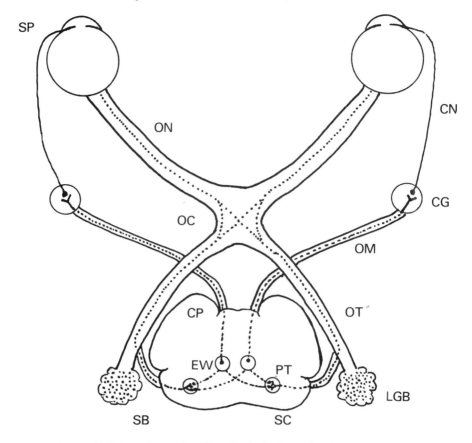

Fig. 5.11   The pupil light reflex paths. The classical schematic view.

CG	Ciliary ganglion		**OM**	Oculomotor nerve
CN	Short ciliary nerve		**OT**	Optic tract
CP	Cerebral peduncle		**PT**	Pretectal nucleus
EW	Edinger Westphal nucleus		**SB**	Superior brachium
LGB	Lateral geniculate body		**SC**	Superior colliculus
OC	Optic chiasma		**SP**	Sphincter pupillae

most simple abnormalities of pupil reactions. The author's own 'aide memoire' is reproduced in Fig. 5.11 for the convenience of the reader.

A reduction or absence of pupillary reaction to light while a normal near response is present is a hallmark of neurosyphilis. Thankfully, this is becoming less common than once was the case for a number of medical and social reasons. If such pupillary reactions are detected, it is probably best not to remark upon the fact directly to the patient; there are some other rare disorders which can also cause near-light dissociation. The patient should be referred to his or her general medical practitioner.

The possibility of mechanical restriction of the iris should never be forgotten; posterior synechiae can sometimes make a pupil appear unreactive, until the iris is more closely observed, using the slit-lamp microscope. Readers should not need reminding that both acute glaucoma and anterior uveitis can also cause a loss of pupillary reactions. A recording of the pupil reactions should be concise and clear, for example:

P.A.,D.C. & N.,B.E.,

states that the pupils are active to direct, consensual and near stimulation in both eyes.

(The author dislikes the American method of recording pupil reactions, viz. 'PERLA — pupils equally reactive to light and accommodation'.)

If an anomaly of pupil size, position or function is found ask the patient whether he or she had any knowledge of the problem. Sometimes the patient can be remarkably well informed about such things, making comments like: 'I've got an Adie-Homes pupil in the right eye.' Any anomalies should be noted. An anomaly of structure or position of the pupil may be more usefully recorded either in the section on the cornea and anterior chamber, or under ophthalmoscopy.

5.8   Motility

The ocular motility should be tested using as small a fixation target as the patient can reasonably see. Unless the patient is partially sighted, a pen torch should not be used unless the practitioner wishes to try and observe the corneal reflexes during the routine. In general, a small fixation target will encourage the patient to fixate accurately, and small degrees of diplopia will be more easily noticed by the patient.

Unless the patient has a refractive strabismus, the motility should be assessed without the spectacles in place, so as to enable to optometrist to see the ocular movements more easily. It is important to illuminate the patient's face adequately during this procedure, as subtle irregularities of motility may be difficult (if not impossible) to detect in poor light.

(The author uses a small white ball, approximately 3 mm in diameter mounted on a black pencil as a fixation target for most of his patients. A drawing of this is shown in Fig. 5.12.)

The patient should be made to keep the head still, and then to follow the target with the eyes, reporting any strain or doubling of the target. The target should then be moved in the six cardinal directions, (see Fig. 5.13) curving the target path around an imaginary centre between the patient's eyes. This curving of the path minimizes the possibility of the optometrist detecting a false anomaly due to variation in fixation distances. The speed at which the target is moved will, to some extent, depend upon the patient's accuracy of fixation and co-operation.

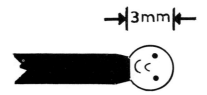

Fig. 5.12 Fixation target on black wand. A 3 mm diameter bead, suitably inscribed, is used on the end of a black wand or pencil some 160 mm long.

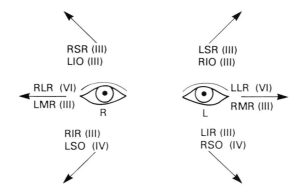

Fig. 5.13 Extra-ocular muscles' main actions and innervations. This aide memoire is useful when limitation of movement of one eye is noticed, also when diplopic images are investigated with a light and coloured filters.

However, a complete 'sweep' of one meridian should take about four to five seconds. Faster movement of the target can lead to a loss of fixation, and an inaccurate result being obtained.

Any failures of extra-ocular muscle action, or abnormalities such as nystagmus, should be noted. Where there is an obvious incomitancy, a tentative diagnosis may be made, but further tests may be needed to establish the exact cause. Any concomitancy should be measured as accurately as possible when the cover test is carried out.

5.9　　Convergence

This should be tested immediately after the assessment of the ocular motility, with the same fixation target. As with the motility tests, the patient should be encouraged to maintain a stable head position, reporting any doubling of the target. It is worthwhile emphasizing that the patient may not be able to see the target clearly as it gets closer to the face. Blurring of the target is not doubling; it is the doubling which should be reported.

There are two main convergence functions which should be checked; Jump and tracking or pursuit. A patient may be able to follow the fixation target up to the tip of his or her nose reasonably easily, but may be quite unable to look directly from a distant target to a near one. This can sometimes indicate a weakness in the appreciation of physiological diplopia, and may be investigated further using 'phys. dip.' techniques.

Both the objective and subjective near points of convergence should be noted, as should the dominant eye, whether the patient appreciated diplopia, or if one eye suppressed the diplopic image.

For example, the notes for a patient with a 12 cm near point of convergence, after which the left eye diverged and produced a diplopic image should read:

N.P.C. 12 cm. L.E.Div + dip.

5.10   Cover test

The cover test is probably the easiest optometric technique to perform, but one of the more difficult to interpret correctly. The inexperienced optometrist can practise assessment of ocular movement by watching a friend look at points separated by a known gap at a known distance. For example, if the target distance is 3 metres, then each 3 cm separation of fixation points gives an ocular movement equivalent to 1 prism dioptre. Thus, having the friend look from the marker to a point 9 cm away from it will produce a 3 prism dioptre movement. When the optometrist has gained experience and confidence in assessing the movements, the friend can be asked to look from the marker to any of the other points used, and allow the optometrist to 'guess' the degree of movement. A few short sessions of this type of practice is definitely worthwhile for any practitioner who needs to improve skill with the cover test.

The author prefers to leave the cover test until this stage in the routine, so that any disruption of binocularity will not adversely affect other tests such as motility or convergence.

The cover test should be used on all patients with two functioning eyes. When a patient wears spectacles, these should initially be worn for the test. Having determined the oculomotor balance with the correction in place, the tests can be repeated without the spectacles. However, little useful information will be gained by carrying out the cover test on an uncorrected highly myopic or aphakic patient.

The cover test should be carried out for at least two viewing distances: six metres, and the patient's habitual near vision position. With some occupations, such as computer users, librarians, and airline pilots, the cover test may need to be performed with the patient looking upwards to simulate their occupational requirements. The fixation target should be appropriate to the patient's visual abilities. Good lighting is essential if small ocular movements are to be detected.

The patient's face should be well illuminated, with as few shadows as possible. (Don't, however, give the patient the impression that you are about to perform an interrogation technique learned from the more unpleasant 'cop' movies! If a direct light, such as an adjustable lamp is used, it should not be too close to the patient's face.)

Patients may occasionally comment on apparent target movement during the cover test. They should be reassured that this is normal, and indeed expected.

The results of the cover test should be recorded concisely, using standard orthoptic notation. The standard unit of measurement is the prism dioptre (pd or $^\triangle$), and use of any other unit is strongly discouraged. The commonly used abbreviations are tabulated below, and an example is given.

XOP	Exophoria
SOP	Esophoria
XOT	Exotropia
SOT	Esotropia
RH	Right hyperphoria
LH	Left hyperphoria

Where a 5 pd left esotropia is found at distance, it may be recorded thus:

CT (d) $5^\triangle$ LSOT -o-

Where a horizontal tropia is detected, the appropriate abbreviation should be prefixed by L or R as required. Where a vertical tropia is detected, it is probably best to record the findings in an unabbreviated mode, to avoid any confusion. A note should also be made of any incomitancy detected, in conjunction with the ocular motility tests.

5.11 Visual fields: central and peripheral

Routine assessment of visual fields has become increasingly automated over the past fifteen years. However, many consulting rooms still have little easy-to-use instrumentation for visual field examination.

A small (3 mm diameter) white map-pin, mounted on a black-painted length of 5 mm dowelling (or a black pencil) is a most useful tool for initial estimation of both central and peripheral visual fields. The author uses the same instrument for this section as for the motility and convergence test.

The practitioner should be seated directly in front of and facing the patient at a distance of about 50 cm. The patient should be asked to cover the eye not being tested, and asked to indicate, either verbally or with a movement of the free hand, when the target is first seen. The patient should be asked to look carefully at either the optometrist's eye or nose, and the target should be gradually brought round from behind the patient's head in an arc centred on the eye being tested, at about

40 cm from the patient's head. The target should be brought in along horizontal, vertical and oblique directions thus giving eight meridians tested.

The central visual field, including the position and size of the blind spot can then be checked by comparing it with that of the optometrist in a direct confrontational fashion. Checking the blind spot will give the practitioner some idea as to the reliability of the patient's responses.

Any loss of field should be recorded giving detail of position and extent of the defect. A note about the patient's reactions can also be useful.

There is, of course, no substitute for accurate central visual field assessment using instruments such as the Friedmann Visual Field Analyser, or the Henson Central Field Screener. The Bjerrum screen, when used by a skilled and experienced practitioner, can also be an accurate and rapid way of examining the central visual fields. Similarly, peripheral field analysis can only be carried out with a high degree of accuracy using a bowl perimeter. However, using such instruments could be considered as being part of supplementary techniques, and will not be considered here.

5.12 Colour vision

Colour vision frequently seems to be a 'poor relation' when compared with other optometric techniques. Perhaps this is because there is rarely any income generated from testing colour vision, (possibly because the provision of advice about colour vision problems has never been properly organized by the optometric profession at large) and such anomalies are rarely caused by sight-threatening conditions. However, as the profession of optometry becomes threatened by auto-refractors and unregistered dispensing, areas previously considered as outside day-to-day optometry may become more important when considering services with which to attract potential patients.

The assessment of basic colour vision is simple, and several excellent tests are available for consulting room use. The most commonly used test is the Ishihara pseudo-isochromatic plates. This is very sensitive, but gives little indication as to actual type or severity of any defect, and it has no plates specifically for testing for tritanopic defects. The City University Colour Vision Test (Keeler Ltd) is more useful when determining the type and severity of defect, and in the Mk 2 version is quite sensitive to mild problems, and both Mk 1 and Mk 2 are designed to detect tritanopic defects. Both these tests are designed to be used under specific illumination; either north daylight, or standard illuminant C.

The Simplified Colour Vision Test (Keeler Ltd) (see Fig. 5.14) is excellent for use when screening children, as it is washable, and designed to be used under tungsten bulb illumination, which is nearly always readily available. It, too, tests for all three types of defects.

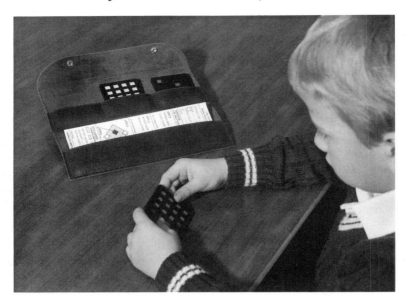

Fig. 5.14 Colour vision test for child or adult. The Fletcher-Hamblin Simplified Colour Vision Test (Keeler Ltd) uses plastics mosaics, ideally under ordinary tungsten light. This provides a rapid test for 'significant' degrees of inherited and acquired colour vision deficiency, whether red/green or tritan. (Courtesy of Keeler Ltd)

A lantern test has special value as a quick and realistic demonstration (to both patient and parents) of errors. In any area where there are sea-faring communities, this test may be particularly appropriate, as the Board of Trade and the Royal Navy still use this type of test.

There are several other colour vision tests available, but this text is not just a catalogue!

In the context of a routine eye examination, all patients should have their colour vision tested either at their first visit to a practice, or (in the case of infants) when they are sufficiently mature to respond accurately. Thereafter, colour vision should be checked whenever there is a pronounced change in either the refraction or the visual acuity, in case there is a pathological cause. Colour perception should be checked monocularly as there are frequently differences between the eyes due to a variety of causes, the most common of which is a difference of light transmission of the ocular media of the two eyes. This can be especially marked in a patient with unilateral aphakia, where the aphakic eye will 'see the world' with a distinctly blue tint compared to the phakic eye. If a patient with two apparently normal eyes exhibits a marked difference in colour vision between the eyes, the possibility of retinal trauma or optic nerve damage should be considered. The normal ageing of the eye, as has already been hinted, affects colour perception. The fact that a patient is over 60 years old should not stop the optometrist checking his or her colour vision. Indeed, some senior citizens need good colour perception to be able to distinguish between different pills and tablets which they may have to take.

If an anomaly is found, it should be classified for type and severity as much as is possible, and the patient should be asked about any family history of colour vision defects. On the subject of communicating with the patient, the term 'colour blind' should only be used for true monochromats. Young people can feel frightened by 'colour blindness', and it is a very negative term to use. If a mild defect is detected, calling it 'Daltonism' (and explaining why) helps the patient to accept it as an altered state of normality rather than as something bad and to be hidden away. The optometrist should not be afraid of giving advice concerning the problems (either in terms of career or hobbies) which colour vision anomalies can cause a patient, although in the case of young males with specific careers as a target, this needs to be done with tact and sensitivity, and sometimes the parent(s) should be counselled first, out of earshot of the patient.

The optometrist should be prepared to prescribe palliative tints, as this form of therapy can be of significant help to a Daltonic patient. This topic is excellently covered by Fletcher and Voke (1985).

Chapter 6
Ophthalmoscopy

6.1   Review of procedures

Ophthalmoscopy is one of the most useful clinical techniques available to the optometrist, and is hence probably the most important single part of the eye examination. Some practitioners like to carry out ophthalmoscopy at this stage of the eye examination, i.e. before the refraction starts. The author's preference is to leave ophthalmoscopy until after the refraction and any specialized examinations which might be affected by having a bright light shone into the patient's eyes (such as colour vision, contrast sensitivity, and central visual field analysis). The author also feels that leaving ophthalmoscopy until the end of the eye examination allows the patient more time to develop confidence in the optometrist. This should reduce any worry which the patient might feel when the optometrist gets close to the patient's face having darkened the consulting room. This is especially true for young patients who may have various fears about the dark which to some adults are irrational.

Ophthalmoscopy can be used for (albeit not very accurate) objective refraction as well as for the detection of any intra-ocular abnormalities.

The patient should be advised that the room lights will be partially or fully (according to the preference of the optometrist) extinguished and a bright light will be shone into their eyes to allow the optometrist to check on the health of the eyes. A suitable fixation target should be chosen, and the patient asked to look straight at it. The target chosen should be easily visible when the room lights have been put out, without compromising the general darkness of the consulting room. It should be in such a position that it can be easily seen by the patient while ophthalmoscopy is in progress. The spotlight on the test chart can be an ideal target, although it may be too low for securing the best fixation direction, depending on the layout of the consulting room and the type of test chart used. Optometrists using a new consulting room should always experiment with different fixation targets until a suitable one is found. The fact that the 'top right-hand corner' is the preferred fixation point in one consulting room does not mean that it will be correct in another.

The patient should be asked to keep the head still, and if necessary it should be gently positioned correctly to allow ophthalmoscopy to be carried out without danger to the optometrist's spine. Sometimes the patient's head may need to be stabilized by the optometrist using his free hand.

It is important to avoid any grunts or other utterances during ophthalmoscopy, unless asking the patient to look in a particular direction. A gasp, or a quiet 'hmmm' when looking into a patient's eye can convince them that their worst dreams of impending blindness are about to be confirmed. Early in the author's career he was forced to spend a considerable time reassuring one lady patient that he was simply breathing in with rather more volume than usual, and had not found a sight-threatening lesion during ophthalmoscopy.

The patient should be allowed to have a rest as often as it seems necessary; patients will naturally vary in their ability to concentrate on a fixation target, and in their tolerance to the bright ophthalmoscope light. Any indication of stress should prompt the practitioner to check the comfort of the patient.

Initially, a high plus lens, usually about + 14, should be selected for viewing the anterior eye and associated structures. The lids, lashes, conjunctiva, cornea, and canthi can thus be inspected (see Fig. 6.1). The power of the viewing lens should then be gradually reduced to about + 10 to allow examination of the crystalline lens. Only about 20 per cent of the lens can be seen without moving away from the visual axis. It is important to check the periphery of the lens as well

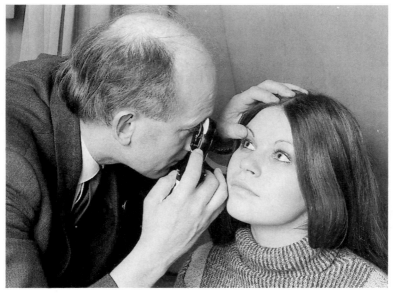

Fig. 6.1 Media examination. The patient fixates initially above the horizontal and extra plus is used to observe the media. Note the thumb holding the upper eyelid, to retract it when the patient looks down. Both hands are being used to steady the position of the ophthalmoscopist.

as the central area, and this can be made easier by asking the patient to look up, right, left, and down as appropriate. Some patients have difficulty in working out in which direction they are supposed to be looking, and in such situations the addition of a comment such as 'towards the door', or 'towards your feet' can be helpful.

Having examined the crystalline lens, the power of the viewing lens in the ophthalmoscope should be gradually reduced, allowing the optometrist to look back through the vitreous gel (checking for any floaters or other artefacts) until the retina is finally brought into focus. It is worth noting that vitreous floaters are often best seen after the eye has been deliberately moved, and to this end, the patient can be requested to 'look straight up and then immediately back to the original target'.

The optic disc is usually the first structure to be identified in the fundus, and is therefore a convenient place to start the examination of the back of the eye. The rest of the central retina should then be viewed. The macula can be viewed either by locating it objectively, or by asking the patient to look directly into the ophthalmoscope light. (If the patient does not have central fixation this technique may not help.) The peripheral areas of the retina can then be examined. This, as the inspection of the periphery of the crystalline lens, requires considerable movement of the ophthalmoscope and also the patient's fixation if a good sight of the extreme retinal periphery is to be obtained. When examining the lower areas of the retina (or the crystalline lens) the patient's upper lid must be lifted slightly to prevent it occluding the optometrist's view. The easiest method of restraining the upper lid is to hold it gently with the thumb of the hand not holding the ophthalmoscope. The rest of the hand can be gently rested on the patient's forehead. Take care not to rest the hand on the patient's hair, as wigs and toupees can easily be thus dislodged, to the embarrassment of both parties.

The experienced optometrist will be able to inspect a fundus and, almost subconsciously, to say whether it appears normal or not, even before attempting to determine what is out of the ordinary. The less-experienced (younger) practitioner should take time to think consciously about the appearance of the fundus and to compare it (mentally at first) with that which is usually regarded as 'normal'. If the optometrist wishes (or needs) to refer to a text book after ophthalmoscopy, the patient is more likely to perceive this as a demonstration of the practitioner's care for them rather than as an indication of incompetence, providing the patient is informed tactfully of the reason for reference. Naturally, it is not a good idea to use emotive words such as 'cataract', 'tumour', or 'growth' when discussing the findings with the patient. (Some general medical practitioners also seem to object to optometrists using words which might indicate that a 'diagnosis' has been undertaken, so make sure that you know the prevailing feelings of the medical fraternity in your area before advising patients of findings or writing referral letters.)

A selection of fundus photographs has been included, to highlight some of the points raised above.

Fig. 6.2 shows excavation of the optic disc, the c : d ratio being about 0.5. The vessels appear healthy, and the junctions show no signs of nipping, humping, or deflection. A cilio-retinal artery is present, leaving the disc at 9 o/c.

In Fig. 6.3 a 'crescent' is visible around part of the disc margin, from 12 o/c to 6 o/c. This appearance is more common in myopes due to the lengthening of the globe, which causes stretching of the structures around the back of the globe, and allows the sclera to show past the edge of the retina and choroid. Also of note in this picture are some retinal ripples, or stretch marks, slightly more than a disc diameter below the disc. Such marks are similar to angiod streaks, and again are more common in myopes.

In Fig. 6.4 the disc appears to be swollen. However, the vessels are of normal calibre, and show no significant tortuosity or other signs of raised blood pressure.

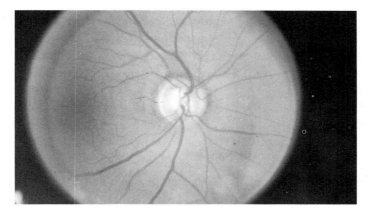

Fig. 6.2

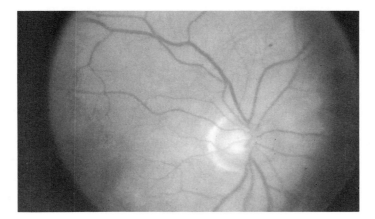

Fig 6.3

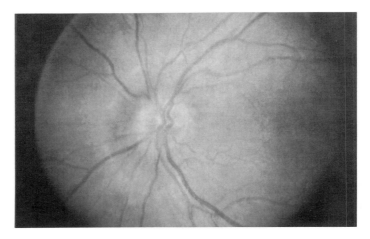

Fig. 6.4

There are no haemorrhages or exudates, and in a symptom-free patient this appearance is pseudopapillitis. The ophthalmoscope can be used to estimate the height of the disc margins above the retinal surface by differential focusing.

In Fig. 6.5 there are many flame haemorrhages present, and the veins appear grossly dilated and tortuous. The arteries appear normal by comparison. This is a case of central vein thrombosis. It is often caused by pressure on the central retinal vein by the central retinal artery at the lamina cribrosa, due to raised blood pressure. Branch vein occlusions have a similar retinal appearance, but it is limited to the sector of the fundus drained by the affected vein.

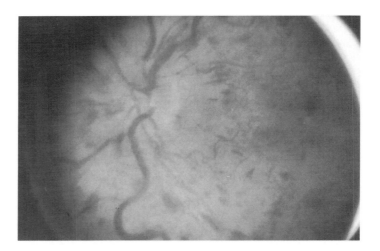

Fig. 6.5

Having carried out a careful inspection of the fundus, any findings should be noted. It is often advisable to complete the recording of findings for one eye before proceeding with ophthalmoscopy of the other.

It is beyond the scope of this text to list all the possible findings during ophthalmoscopy. However, any abnormalities should be carefully recorded, and diagrams are useful. (If a fundus camera is available, so much the better.) The more relevant detail that is recorded, the easier it is to decide whether any change has taken place at a later date.

Use of the expression 'Ophth. N.A.D.' is not really sufficient, as it does not indicate that any particular structure has been examined. Examiners will not be impressed with the use of such terminology, especially in the case records section of the PQEs.

When a problem is encountered viewing the fundus through a small pupil, a mydriatic should be used. The author's drug of choice is 0.5% Tropicamide, which has a relatively rapid action, but short duration, and a minimal effect on accommodation. The normal precautions when using mydriatics should be observed, but practitioners should not avoid using drugs where there is any indication to do so; the risk of precipitating an attack of closed angle glaucoma by the use of a mydriatic or cycloplegic is in all probability vastly less than the chance of missing something important ophthalmoscopically through a small pupil. When using a mydriatic, the IOP should be checked before the drug is instilled, and again after the procedure has been completed, but this is more for protection against frivolous complaint of negligence than for true clinical necessity. The patient should be warned about the possible visual side-effects of a dilated pupil, and some practitioners like to give their patients cards to carry in case of accident or emergency after having had mydriatics used.

If a peripheral lesion is detected, or suspected, then use of an indirect ophthalmoscope is advisable. This will allow (possibly in conjunction with a mydriatic) a better view of the peripheral fundus. The author's preferred instrument is the monocular indirect ophthalmoscope made by Reichert-Jung (American Optical) as it is easy to handle and does not require the use of a separate condensing lens. An indirect ophthalmoscope can also be useful for highly myopic patients, as the degree of magnification of the fundus is significantly reduced. This feature can also assist observation of a moving fundus picture, as in the case of infants, and patients with nystagmus. Binocular indirect ophthalmoscopes, although not initially as simple to use as the direct instruments, have the advantage of providing a stereoscopic picture (providing the optometrist has normal stereopsis) and this can help in the inspection of lesions which are suspected of being raised.

Having completed ophthalmoscopy of both eyes, any particular findings may be discussed with the patient, and any further investigations carried out as indicated (see Figs. 6.6 and 6.7). If there is no sign of any abnormality, the patient

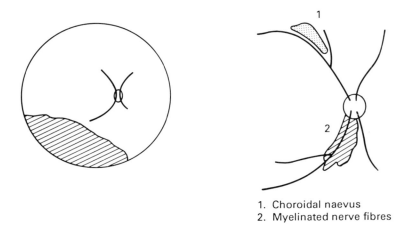

1. Choroidal naevus
2. Myelinated nerve fibres

Fig. 6.6 Sketches on record   (a) To indicate an area of retinal detachment   (b) to indicate choroidal naevus and myelinated nerve fibres.

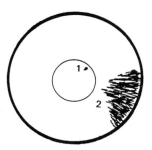

1. Posterior lenticular hyaloid remnant at 2 o/c.
2. Peripheral cuneiform (lenticular) opacities.

Fig. 6.7 Sketches of lenticular opacities. A hyaloid remnant has been located on the posterior capsule and a peripheral cuneiform opacity. Is the former usually as high and is the latter usually temporal or nasal?

may be suitably reassured, remembering that this section of the eye examination can be the most worrying for the patient.

6.2   Ophthalmoscopy 'from the front'

Starting 'at the front', the lids, lashes, bulbar conjunctiva, and adnexa (caruncle, plica etc.) should be examined, paying particular attention to position, size and colour. The tear film can also be assessed by looking at the tear 'prism' along the lower lid margin. These areas have already been covered in previous sections, so the advice and comments will not be repeated here.

The cornea should then be examined for any opacities or irregularities, paying particular attention to the 'lustre' of the surface. The optometrist may already suspect a problem in the cornea if signs of an anomaly have been found during the external examination, (for example, an irregularity of curvature or scarring) or if the patient has recently removed hard contact lenses. Areas of corneal irregularity, either of transparency or surface shape, can most easily be detected as shadows or distortions in the red reflex from the fundus. Corneal dystrophies (epithelial, stromal, and endothelial) can cause the fundus reflex to appear 'grainy', and a poor or irregular tear film can give rise to a wavy fundus reflex. Debris in the tear film can sometimes be mistaken for particulate matter in the anterior chamber; watching how the particles move after blinking should aid determination of location.

The aqueous and anterior chamber are the next structures which come into view, although in a normal healthy eye there will be nothing to see between the cornea and the anterior surfaces of the iris and lens. If particles are detected in the anterior chamber, slit-lamp microscopy is mandatory to check for aqueous flare, and keratic precipitates, in case the patient is suffering from anterior uveitis.

Having examined the cornea and checked the clarity of the aqueous, the iris can be examined. The chapter on the external examination has already covered this structure with respect to its examination with a hand slit-lamp. The use of an ophthalmoscope allows greater magnification of the iris, and if there is any thinning of the iris due to damage, disease, or development, then the fundus reflex may be seen through the atrophic layers of iris tissue (providing there is no dense opacity in the crystalline lens blocking the fundus reflex). (Michelson's *Colour Atlas of Uveitis Diagnosis* has many splendid pictures of such conditions.)

The crystalline lens is the next structure in the pathway, and is perhaps second only to the fundus in ophthalmoscopic importance. There are a variety of 'normal' artefacts which may be observed, such as epicapsular stars, and posterior lenticular hyaloid remnants. Any areas of opacity or haze within the crystalline lens can be located with reference to the pupil plane and/or the corneal reflex (first Purkinje image) which is situated at the approximate position of the back surface of the lens. The location of the artefact can be quite accurately determined by the optometrist, using simple parallax between it and either or both of the two reference positions. For example, a spot of pigment on the anterior surface of the lens will show hardly any movement with respect to the iris, but will move 'against' the corneal reflex when the optometrist moves the ophthalmoscope (see Figs 6.8 and 6.9). When the periphery of the lens is inspected, a difference in the brightness of the fundus reflex in different areas of the pupil should alert the practitioner to the possibility of irregularities in the refractive index of the lens, such as that caused by nuclear sclerosis. In patients over 60 years old, some

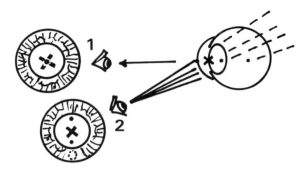

Fig. 6.8 Parallactic displacement relative to pupil. Holding the ophthalmoscope at position 1 lines up four opacities, apparently all central in the pupil. Observation from position 2 shows apparent displacement, relative to the pupil, apart from the anterior lenticular opacity. The deep lecticular opacity appears to move downwards while the opacity behind the lens becomes hidden by the iris. What is the apparent shift of the corneal opacity?

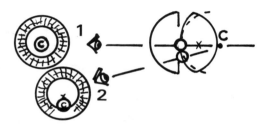

Fig. 6.9 Parallactic displacement relative to the posterior pole on the lens. This relies on the situation of the centre of corneal curvature (c) being near the posterior pole of the crystalline lens. The first Purkinje images, seen from different directions lie on a locus shown as a line of dashes. Observing from position 1 an opacity at C and one at X both appear in line with the Purkinje image O. From position 2, X is seen to be displaced from the reflection but C remains in the same position relative to the reflection.

nuclear sclerosis should be expected, but determination of an acceptable degree is a qualitative judgement, and a matter of experience rather than hard and fast rules (see Fig. 6.10).

The author uses four grades when recording nuclear sclerosis: very slight, mild, moderate, and severe. Most opacities which commonly accompany normal ageing (excepting the already mentioned nuclear sclerosis) start in the peripheral cortex of the lens, and subsequently spread inwards. When recording any areas of relative or absolute loss of transparency of the lens, the diagram should take the form of two concentric circles, the outer representing the edge of the lens, and the inner representing the pupil margin. This will prevent any ambiguity as to the position and extent of the artefact. If appropriate, a cross sectional diagram of the lens can also be drawn. The slit-lamp microscope should be used to examine any

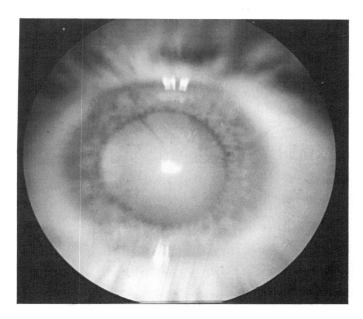

Fig. 6.10 Lens opacities. Although these commencing opacities resemble many senile changes they are here present in a patient little more than 30 years of age, as an inherited condition which is slowly progressing.

opacities detected, as observation under direct illumination can be of significant help in determining their type. For example, 'Blue Dot' cataracts will appear as dust within the lens cortex when viewed with the ophthalmoscope against the fundus reflex, but when the slit-lamp microscope is used the full beauty of their colour becomes manifest.

The vitreous body, while constituting the bulk of the ocular contents, is rarely given much consideration during ophthalmoscopy, unless there are any opacities present. The most commonly encountered opacities are 'floaters', which can be divided into two broad categories: congenital and acquired. The congenital floaters are usually remnants of the hyaloid vasculature, and are generally found in the central vitreous. The acquired opacities can be due to pathological changes within the vitreous body itself (asteroid hyalitis, synchesis scintillans), or due to lesions or diseases of or affecting the retina or underlying structures (haemorrhages into the vitreous due to hypertension, diabetes, etc., white blood cells in the vitreous due to inflammatory conditions such as chorio-retinitis).

In myopes, the vitreous body is generally less solid than in hypermetropes. This is usually due to the increased volume which the vitreous has to occupy in myopes. For this reason, floaters are more mobile in myopes and are therefore more frequently subjectively noticed. Conditions such as vitreous detachment and retinal detachment are also more common in myopic patients. The vitreous body also tends to become more liquefied with age, and this can also lead to predictable symptoms.

After the 'transparent' media have been examined, the practitioner can start the inspection of the retina and associated structures. Usually the first structure to be seen is the disc, which is the intra-ocular portion of the optic nerve. It is about 1.5 mm in diameter, and is slightly vertically oval (often on account of with the

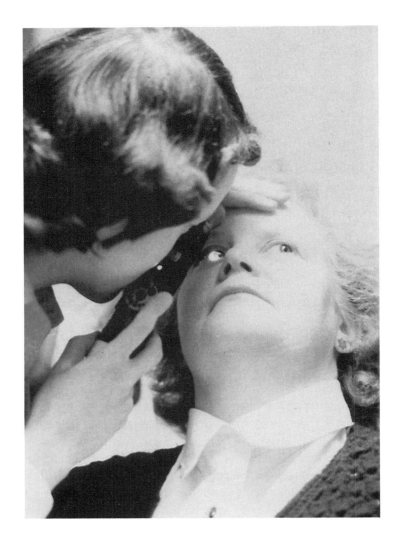

Fig. 6.11 Ophthalmoscopy of the fundus periphery. Note the extreme movement of the patient's eye and the way the brow of the optometrist is rested on the hand for stability.

rule astigmatism). It is situated about 1 mm superiorly and 4 mm nasally to the fovea. The optic disc has many variations of 'normal', and these cannot all be mentioned here, but the important factors to note are its size, colour, cupping, vasculature, and pigmentation. Vascular anomalies, such as cilio-retinal arteries,

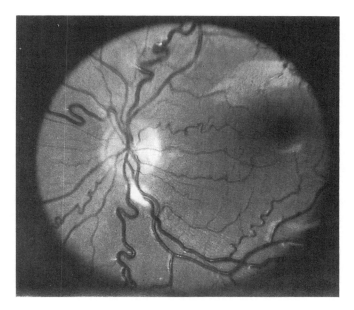

Fig. 6.12 Congenital tortuosity of retinal vessels. Taken in red-free (green) light this photograph by the late E. F. Fincham shows normal but unusual variation in the courses of the vessels. Above the macula the light area is one of the fundus reflections. What is unusual about the region below the lower margin of the disc? In fact, this normal patient has a small area of opaque nerve fibres there.

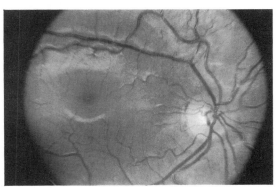

Fig. 6.13 Fundus photo of a young subject. There are extensive reflections, as the fundus 'glistens healthily'. Such reflexes are highly mobile as the ophthalmoscope is moved. Note the appearance of the region around the macula, the foveal reflex and the dispositions of the central vessels. (Photograph by the late E. F. Fincham)

'myopic' crescents, pigment crescents, and any 'veils' of glial tissue overlying the disc, while not usually being of any pathological significance, should be noted. Cupping should be recorded as a decimal proportion rather than as a fraction, and if there is any appreciable difference between the horizontal and vertical cupping, this should also be noted. Cupping of the optic disc is often of no pathological significance, but any disc exhibiting a c : d ratio of more than 0.5 should be regarded as suspicious, and should prompt further investigation. The depth of the cup, visibility of the lamina cribrosa, presence (or absence) of fine vessels within the cup, colour of the neural rim, and pattern of the blood vessels as they emerge from the disc can all help the optometrist to decide whether or not a disc appears normal. (Kritzinger and Beaumont's *Colour Atlas of Optic Disc Abnormalities* (1987) is an excellent book, and should have a place in every practice library.)

Having inspected the disc, ensuring that any abnormalities, or even altered states of normality have been noted, the practitioner can proceed to check the rest of the fundus. This can be done in several fashions: spirally outwards from the disc (preferred by the author), by following the course of the major blood vessels, or by inspecting backwards and forwards along a star pattern from the disc (see Fig. 6.11). The texture, vasculature, pigmentation, and regularity of level of the fundus should all be checked. Retinal pigmentation can vary considerably between even patients of the same racial origin and general complexion.

In general, Asiatic and negroid patients will have darker and often more profuse retinal pigmentation than, for example, a patient with nordic background. Albino patients present a particularly interesting fundus picture, as there is no retinal pigmentation, and the choroidal vessels can be seen underlying the retina. The state of the retinal blood vessels should be noted, paying particular attention to their course, the regularity of the reflexes, their calibre (relative and absolute), and their crossings. While a small degree of nipping can be regarded as normal in a senior citizen, it must be treated as abnormal in a younger patient (see Figs. 6.12 to 6.14).

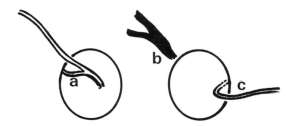

Fig. 6.14 Normal variations of disc region vessels. Which of the three letters refers to (1) a chorio-vaginal vein, which is deeper than the retina and without a reflex; (2) a cilio-retinal artery, usually directed towards the macula (see Kritzinger & Beaumont, 1987); (3) a retino-ciliary vein (or artery); (4) a vessel sometimes also called 'optico-ciliary'?   *Answers:* (1) b; (2) c; (3) and (4) both (a).

Chapter 7
Referral Letters

When an abnormality of structure or function of the visual system is detected during an eye examination, the optometrist is obliged by law to refer the patient to his or her general medical practitioner, or, in the case of an emergency, to the nearest hospital eye department or casualty department.

The referral letter can take several forms, depending largely upon the taste of the referring practitioner

The National Health Service (General Ophthalmic Services) form GOS 18 is probably the most frequently used form of referral letter, and all readers should be familiar with it. Its format encourages brevity and only allows a small amount of information to be included.

Letters which are verbose and unstructured are difficult to read, so many practitioners use a form of 'template' letter which allows the information relevant to the case to be recorded in a logical and easy-to-read manner. This form of letter lends itself to computerization or word processing very well.

Some examples of referral letters are given below. (The usual headings of practice name and address, GP's name and address, and patient's personal details have been excluded.)

7.1   How not to do it!

Dear Dr Smith,

This dear old lady came to see me today for a sight test. She said that she was in good health, and got 6/6 vision in both eyes when I refracted her, although she complained that the sight in her left eye didn't seem as bright as her right eye. Ophthalmoscopy NAD. I can't find anything to explain her problems of headaches, so wonder if you wish to check her over?

Yours sincerely etc. . .

7.2   How it should be done

Dear Dr Smith

Mrs X consulted me today for a routine eye examination. She complains of frontal headaches with no visual association but more marked in the early mornings, for the past four months. Her eyes appear healthy externally, with full motility and good convergence. Her refraction is unchanged since her last examination two years ago, and she achieves 6/6 in each eye. Oculomotor balance, colour vision and stereopsis are all within normal limits.

Ophthalmoscopy reveals clear media, but the discs are cupped (c:d ratio 0.8 in both eyes) and there is some apparent nasal displacement of the retinal vessels. Central visual field analysis shows enlargement of both blind spots, and the intraocular pressures were 26 mm Hg in each eye at 4.15 p.m. when measured by aplanation tonometry. The anterior chamber angles appeared well open.

I think that the symptoms and results of my examination indicate the presence of chronic open angle glaucoma, and I wonder if you wish to refer Mrs X for an ophthalmological opinion.

Yours sincerely, etc. . . . .

7.3   A 'templated' letter

Dear Dr Smith,

Mrs X consulted me today for a routine eye examination, and my findings are recorded below.

Symptoms: Dull frontal headaches in the mornings for the past four months. No apparent visual association.

Vision: R 6/9 L 6/9

Refraction: R $+1.25/ -0.75 \times 180 = 6/5$ $+1.50$ add $=$ N5
             L $+1.00/ -0.50 \times 170 = 6/5$ $+1.50$ add $=$ N5

Oculomotor balance:
Amplitudes of accommodation: All within
Stereopsis: normal limits
Colour vision:

Aplanation tonometry: R and L 26 mm Hg. at 4.15 pm.

Central visual fields: enlargement of both blind spots (copy of charts enclosed).

Ophthalmoscopy: Media: clear. Fundi: Both discs markedly cupped, c : d

0.8, with nasal displacement of the vessels, otherwise healthy appearance.

Mrs X's symptoms may be connected with the signs present of early chronic open angle glaucoma, and I therefore feel that referral for an ophthalmological opinion is indicated.

If you have any questions regarding this letter, please do not hesistate to contact me.

Yours sincerely, etc. . .

7.4   Summary

The content, and to some extent the format, of referral letters depends upon the recipient. Some GPs don't like optometrists to make even the most tentative suggestion as to the possible cause of a patient's problems, as they see this as 'diagnosis' rather than just detection. Other GPs like to be told what is wrong, and some even like suggestions as to how to manage the patient. The optometrist must acquaint himself with the likes and dislikes of the local GPs (and ophthalmologists) and word letters accordingly.

The referral letter is one of the means of enhancing the standing of professional optometry; care should be taken that it achieves this desired result by writing it in such a way that it allows the person to whom it is addressed to read it easily and understand the reason for the referral. If the letter is handwritten, it is therefore important that the writing is neat and easy to read.

A copy of the referral letter should always be kept, in the form of a carbon copy, photocopy, or second printing when using a computer or word processor. This copy should ideally be attached to or kept with the patient's record card.

Chapter 8
The PQE Routine Section

The 'Routine Examination' section of the Professional Qualifying Examinations lasts for two hours, during which time the candidate will be expected to examine two patients (one presbyopic, the other pre-presbyopic), and have an oral which may cover anything in or resulting from the examination of the two patients. This oral may include a discussion on possible further investigative techniques which may be appropriate to the particular patient. It may also include questions on the further management of the patient, with reference to the courses of action which might be taken (e.g. referral, dispensing, etc.).

Many candidates seem to think that they have to perform every test or routine upon their allotted patient, and should do so in such a fashion that the examiner is overcome with admiration for their ability and convinced of their excellence. This is very far from the case. During the routine section of the PQEs, the examiners are required to ensure that the candidate is 'Fit to practise', as defined in the *Guidelines for Candidates, Supervisors, and Examiners on the Professional Qualifying Examination* booklet published by the British College of Optometrists.

The guidelines booklet, and also the syllabus leaflet should be carefully read by all candidates prior to their preparation for the examinations, and also just before entering the exam room. The examiners are concerned with making sure that a candidate carries out all *relevant* tests in a safe and competent fashion, but does not waste time with irrelevant procedures.

Candidates should not use a technique in the PQEs which they have not used and become competent with beforehand. Candidates who do things 'for show' only show up their own problems! It is regrettable, but true, that some candidates forget some basic tests and methods during their pre-registration year. The more common tests which suffer in this way are digital palpation, and confrontation, although even such basic skills as retinoscopy and ophthalmoscopy occasionally prove to be beyond the ability of some candidates.

Ideally, the candidate should make the most of the pre-registration year, and practise as many techniques and procedures as possible. In the PQE, impressing the examiners should not be the aim; instead, concentrate on the patient. Treating the patient as a distant relative is probably a good guide as to the level of communication and care which is ideal. Some 'patients' are experienced subjects, some are optometry students, and some are complete novices, so thare is no standard way to approach them. The candidate should try to make the patient feel comfortable and relaxed, as if the examination was taking place in the candidate's own consulting room.

It should be stressed that all opinions here are those of the author, and are not those of the British College of Optometrists.

Part 2
Oculo-refractive Techniques
R FLETCHER

Introduction

A comparison of different texts on prescribing for ametropia shows some disagreement; take, for instance books by Cholerton, (1948), Giles (1960), Borish (1975), Bennett and Rabbetts (1984a) and Michaels (1985), in which there is a variety of approach. You may or may not agree with the idea that 'refraction' has altered little since Donders' days. Senior colleagues may ask you to adopt some 'house style', often for speed or to integrate you into a team. Examiners, who should be open minded, have been known to express impatience with 'odd' methods candidates may use, or even ask for a particular technique to be demonstrated.

The approach may have to be fitted to a particular patient so it is wise to be sensitive to helpful suggestions from more experienced optometrists. Above all, try to know what you are doing and why; some patients need brief explanations about what you are doing and a listening examiner often appreciates this, for at least two reasons. Facing the PQE you can't afford to be too unorthodox and there is no time to argue your point of view. Soon you will have watched experienced people enough to have picked up some useful tips and to note some questionable methods to avoid. Balance the delight of hearing a patient tell you 'nobody took this amount of trouble before' against the fatigue you will induce by doing too much. Watch for the patient who fails to grasp what is required, or obviously says what appears to be the expected response; reassure, perhaps explaining that you have 'checked the result two ways' so that any difficulty over a patient's decision has been covered.

In the PQE, as in most practical situations, you have the benefit of both objective and subjective data, even your ophthalmoscopic focal power to guide you. This part of the text does not attempt to be other than selective, even provocative in places. In the final part of the book you will find 'real life' situations, to reinforce what comes in the next few pages. If ideas which are new to you emerge, try to compare them to your existing experience and to relate them to your possible future needs.

Become as familiar as possible with relevant British Standards, which you should be able to consult through libraries. These include BS 3162 and BS 2738. In BS 3521:1962, a wide-ranging glossary, note the 'standard' form for writing a spectacle prescription. For example,

$$R + 1.00/ - 0.75 \times 10.$$

Most optometrists can follow this but many do not use it. In this form the Rx uses 'R' and 'L', also 'BE' but avoids such extra 'safeguards' (beloved by some but thought to be redundant by others) such as 'Sph', 'Cyl', 'DS' and 'DC'. Useful standards have been issued on charts and on dichromatic and dissociation test filters.

Chapter 9
Trial Lenses and Other Matters

9.1   Trial lenses

Objective and subjective refractive 'prescriptions' are determined with lenses or combinations, from which errors can arise, some being cumulative. In a new practice or in an examination, look carefully at what you are expected to use. Trial lenses (see BS 3162) can be found which conform to the Standard in form and/or in power but some show significant departures. The BVP at which you arrive using trial lenses will be influenced by the flat surface (if any) being placed towards or away from the eye, as shown in Fig. 9.1. Oblique astigmatism unexpectedly introduced during retinoscopy or subjective tests may depend on this orientation. In a new practice you can take these precautions:

1   Determine the forms of the trial case lenses. At least some of the plus spheres may be equibiconvex.

2   Decide how best to use the lenses, whether with cyls in front of spheres or at the rear. Consider how to use a focimeter to measure the BVP of some combinations which might give 'trouble'.

3   Check the appropriate vertex powers and centrations of all trial lenses, if you can, expecting some surprises! Then, if necessary, decide how you can remedy the situation tactfully.

Among 215 trial lenses in a new set delivered in 1968 series of faults were reported, including a 3.50D cylinder two degrees off axis, many lenses showing strain, a – 6.00DS lens with a central thickness of 0.6 mm and a + 7.00DS lens with 2.4 mm edge thickness.

The implications, for instance for most prescriptions over about 3D, will be brought home by study of the British Standard itself, by reading an account by Bennett (1960) and following what Bennett and Rabbetts (1984a) wrote on the subject, including 'near vision effectivity'.

You are unlikely to be able to treat yourself to an additive vertex power set but do recognize what it could offer. Bearing in mind that most prescriptions are dispensed in 'bent' form, note the advantages of using strong plus sphere trial lenses as in Fig. 9.1, where the cylinder is toward the eye. Take care to know the implications of using your trial lenses in this way. Would the lens markings be

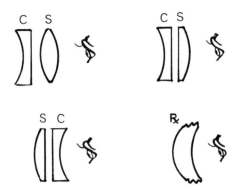

Fig. 9.1 Alternative ways to use trial lenses, compared to the final prescription lens. In most cases the separation between the sphere, S, and the cylinder, C, is not to scale but the vertex distance is the same in all four diagrams. What has to be decided is which form of sphere is in use, where it is placed, relative to the cyl and what are the implications for distance vision, near vision and any resemblance to the performance of the final spectacle lens.

visible? Understand, mentioning in exams where appropriate, the passage in BS 3521 about vertex distances and high powers.

In examinations some 'finer' points may not arise, so in any discussion keep a sense of proportion and avoid a 'know all' attitude. By all means suggest taking the (full) trial frame to a (suitable) focimeter at the end of the subjective tests, having noted the vertex distance, but only in suitable cases. To answer the obvious question 'when is it suitable?' the best action is to experiment a few times, in your practice; then you can speak from experience.

9.2   Refractor 'units' (Phoropters)

These impressive devices use discs of lenses which produce mechanical and optical consequences which are sometimes overlooked. Often such instruments are helpful but not for wriggly children, patients who droop, tilt or retreat behind them or those who insist on 'emerging' for quick comments. I recall a very scientific patient who made an appointment and derided the lack of a 'lens machine' when he was seen by another practitioner. I took care to use a refractor initially, then showed him the need to check the prescription with a trial frame.

Beware of even moderately high as well as near vision corrections prescribed on refraction unit data alone. Note too the possible discrepancies between the 'dial' powers and the BVP of the lens combinations used. Virtually the only way to check such discrepancies is to rig up an *ad hoc* optical bench. Failing all else, read an account by Arden (1951) which should inspire you to serious thoughts!

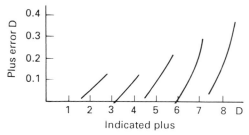

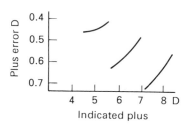

Fig. 9.2 (a) Errors in powers indicated on a refracting unit dial (after Ardern's 1951 data for BRU). Stepped errors are found for a distant object, such that the vergence emerging when the power is supposed to be 7.50DS is about 0.20DS more than indicated by the nominal 7.00DS.

Fig. 9.2 (b) Errors in powers indicated for a near object, also after Ardern (1951). The emergent vergence errors are shown for indicated plus powers from 4.00DS to 8.00DS.

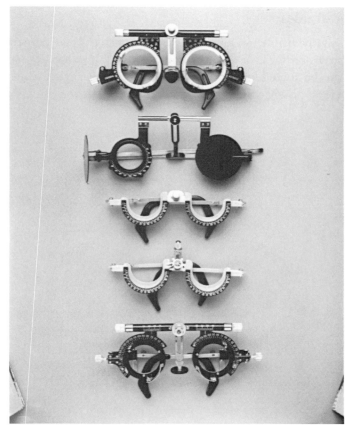

Fig. 9.3 A variety of trial frames. The top and bottom examples permit many adjustments, at the expense of weight. The frame second from the top is ultra light and relies on a single knob for PD and bridge adjustments. (Courtesy of Keeler Ltd.)

Consider the difficulties of binocular near vision testing and prescribing in these situations; one way is to make yourself thoroughly 'hyperopic' with some contact lenses of strong minus power and ask a colleague to treat you as a patient, using the apparatus.

9.3   Virtual lenses in the spectacle plane

A recent and interesting device using the variable power lens systems of Alvarez, projected onto the patient's face, should be noted well. There is now good literature on the matter, including comparative clinical trials and some should be consulted, as well as the price of the apparatus. It would be useful to read the appropriate part of the text by Henson (1983) on this, following up those references which seem to be most useful to you.

9.4   Trial frames

Accurate and highly visible markings, a reasonable range of adjustments, stability, comfort and provision for at least three lenses for each eye are desirable features. Some frames can be angled for depressed visual axes. It is attractive also to be able to measure vertex distances easily or even to slip in low positioned lenses as

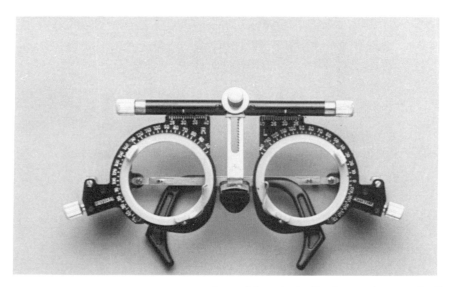

Fig. 9.4 A typical, relatively large aperture frame. Note the inclined control screws for front cell rotation, easy to reach. Sometimes it might be the patient who uses these screws, when axis direction must be checked several ways to overcome uncertainty. What are the advantages of the curved ends of the adjustable sides? (Courtesy of Keeler Ltd.)

'bifocals', but the latter feature is not needed if you have a sensible set of bifocal trial-cum-demonstration lenses (see Figs. 9.3 and 9.4).

If you have a good frame, take it to an examination.

This section closes with a reminiscence. The author took his own trial frame and trial case to the SMC exam but dropped it at the examiner's feet, spilling the contents completely. Without a murmur, the examiner pushed it all under the table, produced another trial set as if by magic and smiled the candidate onward, to a successful examination. So, many of the breed are actually human.

Chapter 10
Objective Refraction

10.1 Retinoscopy

Principles which are well expounded in most visual optics texts should be understood thoroughly and are not repeated here. Rather a number of practical issues will be rehearsed or emphasized.

Certain aspects of this subject arouse prejudices and might do so in examinations. That is, examinations such as the PQE as well as every 'eye examination' you conduct. The choice of retinoscope, the patient's line of sight and possible accommodation are three such matters.

The instrument

Many students are introduced to retinoscopy on model eyes with 'spot' retinoscopes since some teachers believe this to be the best bridge between theory and practice. Usually it is only later, alas, that the advantages of streak retinoscopes are appreciated; by that time a purchase may have been made. What did you first buy?

An ideal retinoscope might be something like that shown in Fig. 10.1. Variable focusing of the beam often helps, in cases with poor media or high errors; also with the help of a suitable plus lens and variable focusing the retinoscope often works well for emergency indirect ophthalmoscopy.

It is obvious that instruments which have interchangeable 'spot' and 'streak' bulbs, even filaments making a right angle, would have advantages. Most practitioners are likely to prefer a streak technique, given the chance.

Instead of a perforated mirror a complete mirror reflecting 40 per cent (or 50 per cent as a second best) of the incident light can be used to good effect, as explained a little later. A variable sight hole size can be provided by a Rekoss disc with holes of perhaps 1.5, 2.5 and 3.5 mm diameter, or an iris diaphragm. An orange filter passes to the patient only such light as will be reflected well from the fundus, reducing glare and usually improving the observer's view. If you have not done so, place such a filter over the projection lens of your own retinoscope. Lee Filters of Central Way, Walworth, Andover, UK can supply small amounts of excellent plastics filters, such as No. 179 'Chrome orange' (Y = 54 per cent, approximately) or No. 104 'Deep amber' (Y = 64 per cent, approximately).

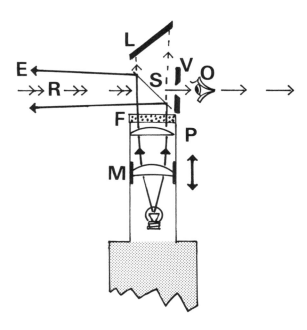

Fig. 10.1 An ideal retinoscope? Light from the streak/spot filament is projected as a divergent emerging beam E, by the projection lens P after suitable change in vergence by the movable lens M. A filter F. orange, red or yellow, reduces the glare to the patient. A beam splitter S allows some light to pass to a light trap, L, which may be black acrylic. The reflected light R from the patient reaches the observer, O, through a variable size sight-hole, V. To what extent does, or could, your retinoscope approach this pattern?

Why irradiate the patient's retina with parts of the spectrum which are absorbed by the fundus? In Fig. 10.2 two possible types of mirror without sight holes are shown. The 10 per cent reflection gives the patient less glare and the retinoscopist less light, as compared to the 50 per cent mirror. Figs 10.2 and 10.3 show the way light is received by both persons, using mirror reflection factors between 10 per cent and 70 per cent, always assuming a 10 per cent fundus reflection, which is only approximate. While the 50 per cent mirror theoretically optimizes matters for the retinoscopist this is at the expense of excess light and a smaller pupil for the patient. A 40 per cent reflection is likely to be the best compromise; 60 per cent would merely penalize the patient.

Act as patient with and without different combinations if you can to appreciate some of these features.

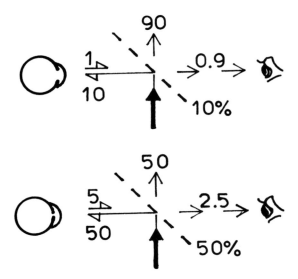

Fig. 10.2 Reflection from non-perforated retinoscope mirrors. Ideas based on views expressed by M. J. Allen of Indiana University. Two situations are shown, one for a glass sheet reflecting about 10 per cent and transmitting some 90 per cent of incident light, ignoring absorption. The other is for a 50/50 reflection/transmission. It is assumed that the fundus reflects 10 per cent of the light it receives, chiefly reflecting red light. Note in which situation both patient and retinoscopist receive more light; this is complicated in practice by pupil diameter changes.

The patient's fixation

Assuming he or she can perform retinoscopy equally well with either eye (and hand) the ideal retinoscopist needs no hair. Absence of ears, a tiny PD and a very narrow skull could be useful. Fig. 10.4(a) suggests the conventional arrangement (beloved by whole generations of examiners) in which the patient fixates a distant (blue ?) object to help accommodation to relax. The patient's 'free' eye might be occluded, particularly if there is a significant 'phoria or squint. Usually the 'free' eye is fogged some 1.50D by initial retinoscopic adjustments on each eye. Hence the ambidextrous optometrist, trained to be ambiocular, 'scopes' the patient's left eye with his left eye. Safir *et al.* (1970) conducted interesting studies, showing 'impressive right-left differences' in precision, using five right-handed retinoscopists. It was noted how discomfort, difficulty in changing lenses, fatigue and awkwardness can result from 'switching observing eyes'; left eyes, usually measured after right eyes, tended to have less accurate retinoscopic prescriptions.

An against the rule astigmatic error is introduced if the angle in Fig. 10.4(b) is more than about 10 prism dioptres. In most cases this could be 'corrected' by

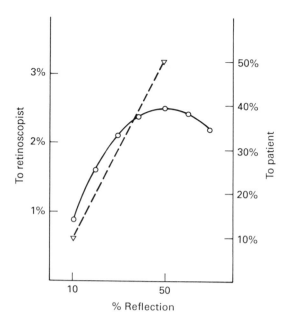

Fig. 10.3 Light which both retinoscopist (circles) and patient (triangles) are likely to receive, according to the reflection properties of the retinoscope mirror. Above 50 per cent reflection, the patient 'suffers' but there is no advantage to the retinoscopist and 40 per cent reflection is a useful compromise. (With acknowledgement to M. J. Allen.)

later subjective techniques, but accurate retinoscopy should be the goal and often it is vital. See Bennett & Rabbetts (1984b).

The common instruction to patients 'look just past my ear' has been criticized to good effect by Hodd (1951). He used an obliquity of between three and four degrees, with two degrees of inferior fixation but changing to some four degrees of lateral fixation gave an apparent relaxation of about 0.25D.

Accommodation during retinoscopy

Fixating an object actually far away tends to relax accommodation. Conversely, knowledge of the proximity of an object, with convergence, stimulates accommodation, despite the 'fogging' of the extra plus required in the compensation for the distance between the retinoscopist and the patient's pupil. A blue distant fixation light in a moderately light room is conducive to relaxation; some use successive fixations, starting from a near object and progressing to a distant object.

Complete darkness can encourage 'night myopia'. Cycloplegia overcomes the potential difficulty and brightens the reflex while spherical aberration becomes more obvious; this seldom lowers accuracy since the central portion of the pupil is easily differentiated. Near reversal the central portion can show a slight relative

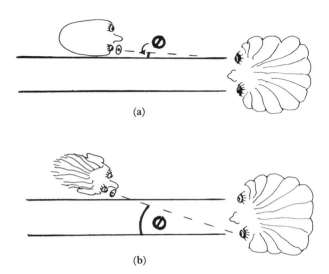

Fig. 10.4 Avoidance of obliquity of view in distance fixation retinoscopy. It is assumed that the patient fixates with both eyes but the retinoscopist always uses the right eye. When observing the patient's right eye the retinoscopist has taken extreme precautions to avoid obscuring the patient's binocular view.

'with' movement, especially if the retinoscopist advances slightly. It is advisable to ensure that both eyes show some 'against' movement early in retinoscopy, before final adjustments. Excessive fogging (over 2.00D) can induce accommodation. Mohindra (1975) introduced a useful dark-room method for children which tends to require more than the usual 1.50DS compensation for working at arm's length. The binocular method of Barratt (1945) has many devotees, who usually end with distant fixation. Some older patients respond well to this method of fixation on an easily seen target on the retinoscope, near the mirror. Astigmatism can sometimes be estimated most accurately if the other eye is occluded.

In the PQE it is wise to use 'conventional' fixation and control of accommodation, ideally after having really mastered the method. Explain any need to depart from this, perhaps because you have an amblyopis eye or an eye injury. Having passed, carefully reassess your techniques and prepare to experiment until you know which method is quick and accurate in your hands.

10.2 Some comparisons

Assuming that subjective refractive data usually overrides retinoscopy, when there is a conflict, you should note any personal bias you seem to produce between the two 'prescriptions'. Artefacts from ocular aberrations and other discrepancies have been summarized by Charman (1975). Numerous comparisons between the two methods have been published. While Safir *et al.* (1970) suggested that an average retinoscopist with an average patient is likely to be within about one dioptre on repeating retinoscopy, it is usual to be more consistent than this. Tolerances for subjective tests will be discussed later but objectively most retinoscopists should expect good agreement with the subjective prescription for astigmatism and only a little more plus sphere by retinoscopy in most cases. Some study of the procedures and results of Freeman and Hodd (1955) is worthwhile. They made repeated independent assessments of some subjects, finding equal facility for arriving at binocular balance, objectively and subjectively.

10.3 Aspects of technique

Sometimes you may be expected to make a record of your retinoscopy as if you had been using only spheres, taking each principal meridian in turn. You may be required to show the 'neutralizing power' for each. Note your working distance. Presumably this convention hopes to avoid doubt about the working distance having been taken into account. It can be encountered in some hospitals.

Since it is tedious to use successive spheres for two meridians at right angles to each other most optometrists use the maximum plus power to neutralize one meridian which leaves an 'against' movement to be dealt with by minus cylinders. Some advocate plus cylinders; a trainee ophthalmologist in the USA once expressed incredulity on hearing the minus cylinder suggested since he had never heard of using other than plus cylinders.

Some simple acquaintance with streak retinoscopy should be of interest if you have not used the method. The same principles are applicable, less easily, to spot instruments. Use an emmetropic model eye or (monocularly) an emmetropic colleague. First obtain 'reversal' with a spherical lens, say + 1.50DS, then deliberately introduce a known astigmatism by placing at + 1.00DC × 160.

1   Focus the streak on a distant wall, then make the beam more divergent. You could use a + 2.000DS temporarily held near the instrument, in the beam, to focus the filament on a wall one metre away to prove that you have a beam diverging 1D.

2   Pretend that you have guessed the power of the required astigmatic correction correctly, as − 1.00DC but believe the axis should be at 180 degrees.

3   Add this − 1.00DC × 180 to the trial frame lenses, then (with the fairly blurred streak image vertical) drive across the patient's face and pupil, along 180°. See Fig. 10.5.

4   Note the direction of the reflex, particularly as you repeat the horizontal drive rapidly. Would you describe it as 'with movement, along a meridian not far from vertical'? Or an 'against' movement?

5   Rotate the streak 90 degress so that it is horizontal on the face, then drive it along 90. Note the direction and type of the reflex movement.

6   Change the axis of the − 1.00DC to 170. Then drive the beam along 170, with the streak orientated along 80; also drive along 80 with the streak lined up with 170. Reflex movements should be interesting. Perhaps you feel they are now more naturally obeying the directions of drive.

7   Capitulate – put the − 1.00DC axis 160 and drive along 160, when you can expect to have 'reversal'. Then drive along 70 (the streak now orientated along 160) and again there should be a neutralization of movement, which you can change to 'with' by advancing, or to 'against' by retreating a little.

If this whets your appetite read one of the detailed accounts, such as written by Freeman and Hodd (1955) or Pascal (1952)

If one principal meridian is neutralized with spherical lenses and a minus cylindrical lens is used to neutralize the other principal meridian but at an incorrect axis, a new (mixed) astigmatic error is introduced. The effect is that of obliquely crossed cylinders. Pascal (1952) applied the term 'guide meridian' to the 'with' meridian produced, at an angle (the guide angle) to the axis of the incorrectly placed minus cylinder. Turning the axis towards the guide meridian and progressively reducing the guide angle produces movements more exactly at right angles to the cylinder axis. This enables the cylinder power to be adjusted, at the correct axis, to neutralize all meridians.

Retinoscopy can be made very difficult by lens opacity and or miosis, when it is often helpful to reduce the working distance, with appropriate modification to the 'allowance'. A very useful approach, described by Carter (1986) (see Fig. 10.6) involves placing a + 5.00DS lens half way between the trial frame and the

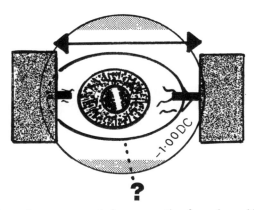

Fig. 10.5   Driving the retinoscope streak image on the face along 180 (see text) with the − 1.00DC axis (incorrectly) at 180, attempting to neutralize the 'refractive error' which really needs the − 1.00DC axis 160. Best understood by following the experiment suggested in the text.

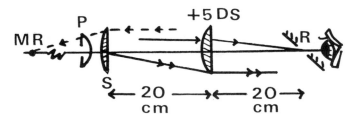

Fig. 10.6 Retinoscopy with a + 5.00DS lens (after Carter 1986). The patient's pupil P is viewed through the neutralizing lenses which are in the spectacle plane S and also the + 5.00DS lens which is placed as shown. The neutralizing lenses in this case focus light from infinity at the patient's far point MR. Parallel light pencils emerging from the patient's pupil via the neutralizing lenses are focused at the sight hole of the retinoscopist R.

retinoscope, which are 40 cm apart. Thus the patient's pupil is significantly magnified, the trial frame lenses at neutralization give the distance prescription, and as Carter suggests, astigmatism can be estimated by moving away from the + 5.00 DS lens since each centimetre of extra distance represents 0.25D.

10.4 Keratometry

While Helmholtz called his device for measuring corneal curvature the 'ophthal-mometer', the alternative name 'keratometer' is usually used today. Measurement of corneal astigmatism has been regularly in use for legal reasons, or for the care of aphakics in some places. However, in the UK in the era 1930–50, few optometrists greatly valued keratometry. Interest in contact lenses rapidly revived the technique, as explained by Fletcher (1955) and Emsley (1963), but still it is unusual to consider the data in 'ordinary' refractive cases. This is often a pity, especially bearing in mind the 'impressiveness' of such a technique and the extra information about the cornea which is gained. As a student I once asked my father if I could practise with his large and always unused keratometer which stood in the consulting room; he said that it had never worked and was retained for appearances, or words to that effect!

Accuracy of measurement of radius can be within 0.02 mm which corresponds to about 0.12D of refractive power, using the refractive index 1.3375 for conversion. This index applies to most but not all keratometers and introduces a compensation for the small (opposite) refractive contribution of the back surface of the cornea. A back surface astigmatism of 0.25D against the rule is likely when the front surface has a with the rule astigmatism of 1.25D. Many eyes are emmetropic because some 0.50D of total corneal astigmatism is cancelled by an equal amount of against the rule lenticular astigmatism. Such practical aspects are

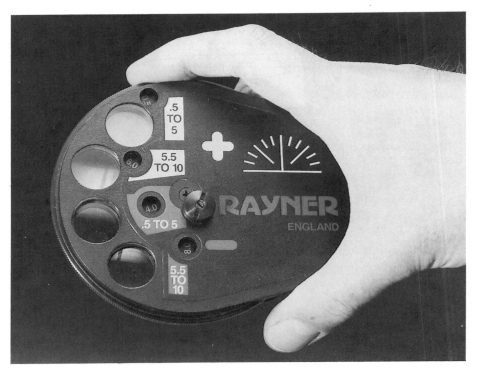

Fig. 10.7   A compact aid for retinoscopy which is a convenient alternative to the conventional rack of lenses and which gives a wide range of powers. How might the effective powers of the stronger lens combinations be determined? (Courtesy of Rayner Optical C.)

apt to be forgotten, when the instrument is chiefly used to find the flattest curve of the front surface as in much contact lens practice.

In practise it is important to ensure that the patient is comfortable, well informed about the purpose and about what he has to do and is fixating well. A blink should be prompted just before a measurement. Use the doubling and focusing devices of the instrument to the best advantage, always adjusting the focus of the eyepiece graticule as a preliminary and using clear, central images of the mires.

Refractive implications

Javal's classical rule can be expressed as

$$\text{Total Spectacle Plane Astig.} + 0.50D = \text{Corneal Astig.} \times 1.25$$

where the modification of 0.50DC represents the non-corneal against the rule astigmatism and is sometimes reduced to 0.25D in youth or raised to 0.75D in the aged.

Thus a keratometric astigmatism of -2.00DC against the rule would be modified to a likely spectacle correction of -2.00 DC against the rule. If the keratometer indicated -2.00DC with the rule, would the spectacle astigmatism be most likely to be zero, -0.75 DC against the rule, -0.75DC with the rule, or -1.50 DC with the rule? According to the proposed scheme described above, the answer should be the last alternative. Various ingenious alternatives to Javal's approach have been suggested and it is likely that the spherical component of the prescription can slightly modify the spectacle place astigmatism.

Estimation of astigmatism in aphakics is particularly well assisted by keratometric readings, which are also a good guide for tracking the changes as healing of the corneal incision progresses. In some operative procedures a portable keratometer is used to dictate the suturing so that the corneal form is optimized. A decision as to when a final, stable, prescription can be issued is most soundly based on such measurements. Corneal irregularity, as in keratoconus, is readily detected by careful keratometry, warning one that a difficult refraction is to be expected.

10.5 Objective optometers

Having developed from subjective optometers, the objective variety passed through one phase in which they were adaptations of ophthalmoscopes, focusing retinal images. Disadvantages included accommodation and the principle was a prey to ocular abberation, snags which have still to be considered in the most up-to-date versions. The real interest for optometrists, who should have some fellow feeling for optometers, has always been how well such instruments perform in practice. One feels sorry for patients seen in tiny Hong Kong cubicles whose prescriptions are dictated by the turn of a switch and the whirr of a printed-out opinion. Performance can be interpreted in different ways, as an expanding literature shows. Now that images are formed by infra-red radiation a wavelength 'correction factor' has been applied to the dioptric scale.

Except as an impressive preliminary, carried out by an assistant, the objective optometer has little to offer the optometrist who can use retinoscopy well. Yet it is worth noting how much stress is placed on the attractiveness of 'computer' or 'automatic' refraction, to which some patients inevitably respond. It resembles the faith placed in gleaming refraction units for subjective use. Note this aspect in McCaghrey's (1989) field trial of seven instruments and the potential advantages when the data is linked with a computer record and or a subjective refraction unit.

McCaghrey stressed the 'significantly different' prescriptions sometimes suggested by different instruments for an individaul. Also to be considered is the likely difficulty when small pupils are encountered or when contact lenses are less than stable.

Every time you go to an exhibition ask different firms, on the same day, to use you as a subject and return to each for a 'second run'. This is frequently most revealing. Griffiths (1988) might well be read for some of the potential snags he mentioned. Nyak *et al.* (1987) compared data obtained with and without cycloplegia. Fletcher (1960) described optometers of the recent past. A detailed exposition of a 'middle generation' of infra-red optometers is to be found in a thesis by Guillon (1978), who showed how most instruments were accurate to about plus or minus 0.50 <d for power and plus or minus 10 degrees for axis. His data on 'repeatability' compared with that of retinoscopy. An important application of the successive analogue records that the Ophthalmetron can produce was shown by Guillon to guide final prescribing for aphakics, when the cornea is settled, usually after about six weeks.

Returning to what impresses patients, the optometrist at every stage of a career might ponder the relative importance placed upon expensive machines or on the skill and care of a pleasant practice. Is the answer completely on the side of mechanization?

Some variations

While considering optometers in this context, mindful of the subjective procedures which are to follow, some bridging can be useful. Subjective optometers have experimental applications and there are 'automated' modern versions. Even simple subjective optometers can be helpful in assessing accommodation (or ametropia) in certain patients with poor VA. Refractive screening, meridian by meridian, has been carried out by laser speckle measurements. This is an interesting but not particularly accurate technique, as Charman and Jennings (1974) showed in a short account. Much the same can be said for optometers which use cortical responses as indications of spectacle prescriptions and for photographic adaptations of retinoscopy.

Most patients and the parents of young patients appreciate brief explanations so that the point of view (sic) of the person who has to use the prescription is usually worthy of serious consideration. The hazards of intolerance of the most theoretically 'correct' spectacles overshadow most of what has been said above, not least when changes in astigmatic correction are indicated or in anisometropia.

Chapter 11
Subjective Techniques

11.1   Correcting spherical ametropia

Few ametropes are completely free of astigmatism but there are some corrections required simply for myopia or hyperopia. The 'best sphere' is an important stage in the correction of astigmatism with astigmatic lenses. Did you ever come across the suggestion in a textbook of ophthalmology, that one procedure for astigmats is actually to prescribe spherical lenses? Presumably it would be better than nothing in some cases!

Estimation of ametropia based on vision

The (unaided) vision of an eye with spherical ametropia often gives a rough guide to the extent of the error. While hyperopes with sufficient accommodation may render the estimate uncertain it is likely to be more accurate in myopia; yet some myopes defeat the prediction since they are used to interpreting blur, or perhaps they narrow their palpebral apertures to gain a line or two on the letter chart. Fig. 11.1 suggests possible estimates for uncorrected ametropia up to about 2 dioptres. Fogging of 1.00DS usually reduces VA of 6/6 to about 6/18 and + 0.50DS usually fogs to about 6/9. Bennett and Rabbetts (1984a) gave a useful compilation and a paper by Swaine (1925) is still worth reading.

In passing, note the possibility of estimating the extent of any astigmatism present, ideally when the 'best sphere' is in place; about double the amount of astigmatism equals the reduction in letter acuity produced by a certain amount of myopia.

The luminance of the chart and pupil diameters are influential, as in all assessments with letter charts.

Monocular sperical correction

Plus spherical lenses are tried first, a power being chosen to overcorrect any expected hyperopia by perhaps one dioptre, thus fogging a little and reducing VA. At this stage the patient is asked whether the lens makes vision worse. The type of question, your tone and expression must all be chosen with care. Convey the

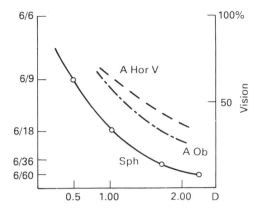

Fig. 11.1 Effects of ametropias on vision. Conditions will cause minor variations from these suggested trends. Full line indicates spherical ametropias, typically myopias. Dotted line indicates oblique astigmatism. Dashes indicate astigmatism with principal meridians horizontal or vertical.

idea that you expect at least the possibility of a certain reaction, without suggesting that it should be inevitable; do not undermine confidence in your knowledge, at least not at this point! Encourage accurate reporting by the patient. Intoning 'better, or worse, or just the same?' with every single lens change is a poor approach. A rash suggestion at any stage would be 'That's better, isn't it?' since it could be met by a flat contradiction. Adapt the size of each lens change to the situation, only using small steps of 0.25D or 0.50D when refining the correction. Anticipate possible accommodation and encourage relaxation by fogging (by up to 2.00DS, no more) and by preventing the patient from viewing the chart without adequate power in front of the eye as you change lenses.

Hyperopes are carefully fogged, with some reassurance that the blur is intentional, after which plus power is reduced in stages, usually retracing the series with an extra + 0.25DS for a slight blurring at the end, when the best VA is reached. Duochrome balancing, then the extra + 0.25DS, can be used at this point.

Myopes are brought to the best VA by increasing minus power in steps, which can be large ones at first. Near the likely end point, ask whether an extra small amount of minus really permits more letters to be read or if 'the letters are just blacker and a little smaller'.

Plus 1.00DS should be added finally, to discover if this blurs the expected amount, usually from 6/6 to 6/18; some relaxation of accommodation may emerge with this fogging. In some cases the slight blur of a smaller excess of plus, 0.50DS or 0.25 can be detected and is informative.

Duochrome

Ocular refractive power depends partly upon the part of the spectrum used, the chromatic aberration of the eye being about 2.00D.

If emmetropia is assumed for light of wavelength 587.6 nm, about 0.50D of myopia would result if 510 nm is used, since the eye has a greater power for this light. Using 750 nm would produce about 0.50D of hyperopia. So if an uncorrected myope of 0.50D views a conventional duochrome chart with letters or circles on both red and green backgrounds he should see the letters 'on red' clearer. A useful aid to memory here is the simple approach shown in Fig. 11.2.

British Standard 3668:1963 briefly explains the use of 570 nm as a 'reference wavelength' when tungsten light is used in a duochrome chart, as is most often the case. Specifications for red and green filters are given so that there is a dioptric difference of about 0.50D between the two positions of clarity. The effective maxima of the respective bands of transmitted light, in practice, become 539 nm and 620 nm. See Bennett (1963) for more details.

Protan observers can use these tests in most cases but the red background will appear to be particularly dark to protanopes, who comprise about 1 per cent of the male population and are worth looking out for. With protan or deutan patients avoid using the colour names but refer to the locations of the respective portions of the chart.

Remember that macular pigment, which varies between individuals, normally provides a physiological filter which reduces the chromatic degradation of retinal images in normal vision; see Walls (1942) and Reading and Weale (1974).

The 0.50D dioptric difference between the two parts of the duochrome test is a wise limit and the widths of the lines of the test objects used are best when between 2 and 4 mm, in fact both sizes are often used. This is because the method is relatively unreliable for uncorrected refractive errors over about one dioptre. Hence the search for the 'best sphere' usually starts with a letter chart with a white background, even if it ends with the duochrome chart. Both young and old patients often accept up to − 0.50DS more by duochrome than they would with careful fogging. In the young you can obtain 'equality', then add + 0.50DS for a

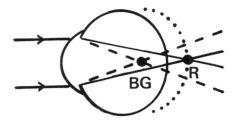

Fig. 11.2 Aide memoire on ocular chromatic aberration. Red light is most in focus for the myopic eye shown in dotted outline. The eye would have to be hyperopic if the best focus were to be for blue-green.

few seconds; ask the patient on which colour the clearer characters appear immediately after you remove this + 0.50DS. See Chapter 19, cases 24–26.

11.2   Occlusion by a plus lens

There are alternatives to opaque occlusion of one eye during the refractive tests on the other eye. Translucent occluders such as ground glass can help a patient to feel less 'lop sided' and may have a small effect on pupil size. While at first this may seem to belong more in section 11.6, where 'balancing' is considered, a technique proposed by Humphriss (1962, for example) has attracted recent attention and will now be described. It involves the binocular effects of lenses related to refining each monocular prescription. There are some advantages, including speed and the ability to check an existing spectacle correction, a tentative prescription or a conventional monocular result.

Humphriss used the term 'immediate contrast' but a succession of comparisons is really involved, asking which of two successive lens situations is preferred. The so-called 'psychological septum', as it is described, relies on binocular vision with relatively similar parafoveal images, a weak monocular fogging lens (+ 0.75 to + 1.00DS) instead of occlusion and concentrates on choices with lens adjustments affecting the non-fogged eye.

It is assumed that accommodation (binocular) relaxes under the fogging and that a significant increase of (binocular) blur is unacceptable if a minus lens tempts the non-fogged eye to accommodate. Thus excess minus (say, – 0.50DS) or plus (say, + 0.25) powers are rejected when the prescription is correct. Crossed cylinder refinement of the prescription is possible with this scheme, provided a minimum of accommodation is encouraged in young patients. The original sequence of lenses (for the non-fogged eye) involved (a) three seconds of + 0.25DS followed by (b) one second of – 0.25DS (called 'test lenses'). Next (c) three seconds of a minus ('moderating') lens is presented, combined with a plus ('test') lens for three seconds; these combine to zero power. Finally (d) the minus 'moderating' lens is retained but a minus 'test' lens is added for one second. The subject at each of the two stages is expected to prefer (b) to (c) and (c) rather than (d).

Meanwhile the fogged eye is regarded as a passive partner at points (a) and (b) and is not expected to detract from (b) being favoured. The point at which (c) is in action leaves the fogging as before but at (d) the fogging increases enough to prompt (c) as preferable to (d). It is useful to try all this and if you find it helpful, note that the + 0.25DS 'test' and – 0.25DS 'moderating' lenses are presented more rapidly in later modifications of the technique; one second and half a second, respectively, are suggested.

Ensure that a single letter rather bigger than the starting VA is used and present the forced choices as which is the 'better' when comparing (a) with (b) and then (c) with (d).

11.3   Crossed cylinder refraction for astigmatism

The elegance and accuracy of other methods, as well as their impressive appeal to some patients, make it difficult sometimes to understand the popularity of the 'cross' cylinder technique. Speed, simplicity and the relative ease with which retinoscopy approximations can be adjusted account for its widespread use. A surprising minority of users does not follow the most logical procedures, as can be seen if you observe several practitioners applying the cross cyl. Best results can be expected when a set of cross cyls is used, with circular test objects of different sizes, rather than letters, since the astigmatic distortions of many letters cause differences in interpretation (Fig. 11.3). Use one lens, + 0.25DS/ – 0.50DC and one + 0.50DS/ – 1.00DC, preferably in small diameters about 30 mm. Two identical sets can be useful. While a lens 1.00DS/ – 2.00DC has some application if you have many patients with very poor VA, some strong astigmatic corrections, above 4D perhaps, are not easy to deal with using a cross cyl.

British and American makers use opposite codes when placing red and white dots or lines on axis/meridian situations and Japanese makers seem to use either (see Fig. 11.4).

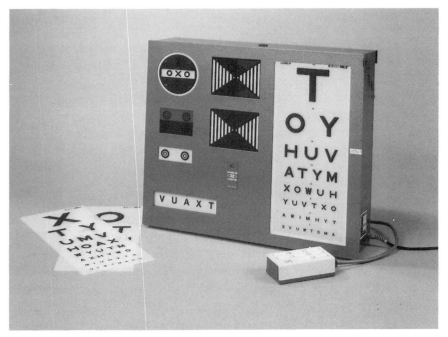

Fig. 11.3   A recently designed internally illuminated chart for wall mounting, with remote control. Can the letter chart shown be used 'direct' and also with a mirror? (Courtesy of Keeler Ltd.)

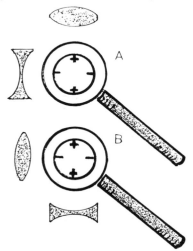

Fig. 11.4 Two alternative X cyl markings. Which would be more likely to be used in the USA? Would the same apply to the UK? Which do you use?

Cross cylinders are useful in retinoscopy, if you need to change the power in one meridian rapidly. Would such use give you the spherical adjustment then required? Many people overlook the principle that the 'circle of least confusion' should be kept on the retina, by adjustments of sphere equal to half any change in cyl power, but of opposite sign. Thus if you have say $-2.50/-2.00 \times 180$ in the trial frame and change the cyl to -1.00×180, you should change the sphere to $-200D$. This adjustment is most important in aphakia or with cycloplegia but it is not wise to neglect it, except when a young patient's minus cyl correction is slightly increased and he or she is able to accommodate 'to provide the extra plus'. Hence young patients are usually given $-0.50DS$ added to the 'best sphere', before the cross cyl is applied, allowing some accommodation to exist. Useful steps are as follows:

1 Obtain the best sphere (e.g. $+1.00DS$)
2 Modify where appropriate, (e.g. to $+0.50DS$ if young)
3 Select a weak cross cyl if the astigmatism is likely to be up to 1.00DC or a stronger cross cyl (at least initially) for higher astigmatism.
4 Seek the cyl axis, tentatively, by placing the cross cyl minus axis first H then V, followed by 45 then 135 and note the two directions most favoured by the patient. Some patients prefer to indicate which, of a pair of positions, is 'better', while others respond most readily by a 'worse' choice.
5 Guided by the preferred direction of the cyl axis, usually a choice between two (e.g. if between H and 45, you would initially put a plano cylinder, say $-0.75DC$, axis 30) go on to provide a tentative astigmatic correction with a minus cyl. What

would be needed then? Yes, an extra plus sphere, half or a little under half the cylinder power change.

6 Modify the sphere, e.g. from the + 0.50DS in step (2) to + 0.75DS.

7 Seek the true minus cyl axis, using the minus cyl axis of the cross cyl first at 75 then at 165 and adjust the plano cyl axis direction. For example if 165 is preferred, the true axis is likely to be nearer to the horizontal than 30, so move it to 25.

8 Repeat (7), using the minus cyl axis of the cross cyl at 70 and 160, that is 45 degrees on each side of the plano cylinder axis you have, until no preference is expressed.

9 Seek the true cyl power needed, using the minus cyl axis of the cross cyl first at 115, then at 25, that is at 90 degrees to the plano cyl axis and parallel to it. Adjust the plano cyl power as required, e.g. if the 25 position is better change the plano cyl to − 1.25DC × 25; naturally, modify the sphere, theoretically to + 1.12DS but in practice to + 1.00DS.

10 Repeat (9) until an end point is reached, with no preference between the two positions of the cross cyl.

11 Ensure that the head and trial frame are level before you finally decide on the cylinder axis required. Consider vertex power factors and the relative positions of the lenses.

12 Repeat steps (7) to (11) whenever necessary.

13 Modify the sphere to best VA.

14 Fog and make any other usual modifications to the sphere.

Note how an extra X cyl + 0.25DS/ − 0.50DC could be held up at step (9) with its − 0.50DC × 25, while the original X cyl is manipulated, to change BOTH sphere and cyl, as a temporary measure (see Fig. 11.5).

Plus cylinders are used by some practitioners, for example when dealing with aphakics or when they wish to write the prescription in the plus cylinder transposition for ordering final lenses, so that clerical errors should be avoided. Provided that suitable spherical changes are made the method is a reasonable one.

11.4 Fan, V and block used with fogging techniques

Apart from the X cylinder there are several approaches to the correction of astigmatism, using different charts. Fogging is employed to maintain control of accommodation and the secret of success is to have the correct relationship between the retina and the different parts of the conoid of Sturm. You could probably manage, at a pinch, using just a pair of lines at right angles, which should rotate simultaneously to any orientation. Or simply a fixed 'fan' of radiating lines, set at ten-degree intervals, could be used.

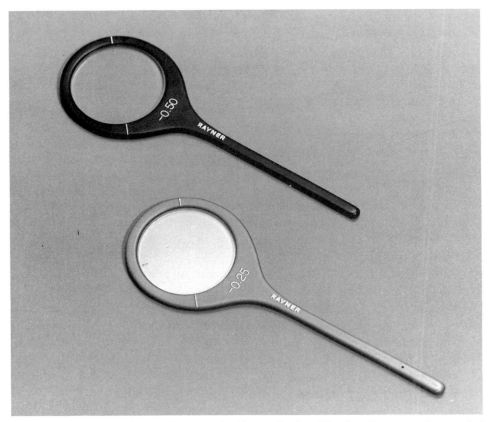

Fig. 11.5 Crossed cylinders in an optimally small size. The handles are colour coded, according to power. (Courtesy of Rayner Optical Co.)

The basis is the control of the positions of the two 'focal lines', the astigmatic images of each point on the test chart. Fig. 11.6 shows how a point object is imaged in with the rule astigmatism which requires a minus cylinder axis horizontal to correct it. When the circle of 'least confusion' is situated on the retina by a 'best sphere' lens, there is little indication as to the direction of the astigmatism and only some indication as to its extent. Adding enough plus sphere to bring the back focal line (in this case the vertical one) onto the retina makes vertical objects clear and indicates the need for a minus cylinder axis horizontal.

Such a 'fogging' plus sphere is extra to the 'best sphere'; it should be equal in power to half the astigmatism. Note some resemblance to the optical features of the cross cyl method, but remember that you do not 'fog' when using the X cyl. The circle of least confusion is always (dioptrally) half way between the two focal lines.

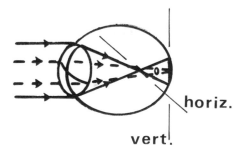

Fig. 11.6 With the rule astigmatism in the eye produces two line images of a distant point object. In this example the simple myopic astigmatism should be corrected by a minus cylinder axis horizontal.

If the point object in Fig. 11.6 is replaced by a fan of lines and the fogging sphere is correct, the patient easily identifies the clearest part of the fan, in this case where the vertical lines are.

To find the exact minus cyl axis required, a rotating V is used, pointing to the 'best line' direction and then being moved until neither limb of the V is clearer than the other. Some rotation from this position of equality, each way, reduces the visibility of the limb which is less correctly orientated at any moment. This is all done with the correct fogging lens in place.

Starting with a minus cylinder power slightly less than the estimated astigmatism, placed at an axis at 90 degrees to the 'best line', as accurately located with the V, you reduce the inequality of the fan lines. This is best done using two 'blocks' of parallel lines set at 90 degrees to each other, with one block parallel to the 'best line' of the fan. Cylinder power is altered until the blocks appear equally clear. The steps are as follows:

1   Obtain the best sphere, using the letter chart (e.g. + 1.00DS).
2   Estimate the amount of astigmatism from the amount that can be seen (e.g. 2.00 of astigmatism, for 6/18).
3   Add a fogging lens, half the estimated astigmatism, always a plus sphere (e.g. an extra + 1.00DS, making + 2.00DS total). See (Fig. 11.7).
4   Locate the best line on the fan (e.g. 90 degrees).
5   Fog a little more (e.g. by holding up + 0.50DS or + 0.75DS extra) to ensure that the best line merely blurs and does not change, in which case your fogging would probably have been insufficient.
6   Reassured, return to the total sphere of + 2.00. If at step (5) the best line did not blur, increase the fogging power until it does.
7   Use the V to locate the meridian exactly at 90 degrees to the required minus cyl axis, that is the exact position of the best fan line, or a direction between two lines.

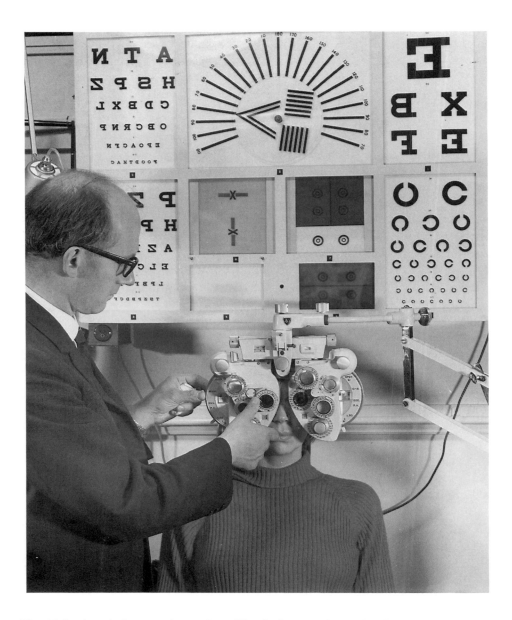

Fig. 11.7 A typical reversed test chart. The fanlines (anticlockwise from the vertical line, which is numbered 180) are numbered 170, 160 and so on, in 10 degree steps. The patient is viewing with a mirror so the horizontal fan lines are numbered 90, to indicate the axis of a minus cylinder correction. Here the double arrow is aimed at a line numbered 80 so a minus cyl axis 80 is required. Provided fogging is correct the cyl power should equalize the two blocks.

8 Equalize the blocks with minus cylinder power, the axis being at 90 degrees to the point of the V.

9 Add + 0.50DS, which should blur both blocks equally. If not, use step (10).

10 Place a plano cyl + 0.50DC, first with its axis parallel to one block, then parallel to the other block. Each block in turn should become clearer, in a logical order, as you first undercorrect then overcorrect the correct minus cylinder. If not retrace your steps fully, with a view to better fogging.

11 Modify the sphere power to best VA, then fog and refine the sphere as usual. All this can be done rapidly, even while you allow the patient plenty of time to answer your simple, direct, questions at each stage. The technique becomes something of a performance, enjoyed by the optometrist and most convincing to the patient as each move progresses to a final clear result!

There are other ways of presenting the test object for fogging. Raubitschek's chart is based on two parts of a parabola or hyperbola, as shown in Fig. 11.8. This replaces the fan, V and blocks, looking like an insect's antennae. The clearest region of one limb is first located, under fogging, when the chart is rotated to equalize the most parallel parts of the two limbs, like the V previously used. Then

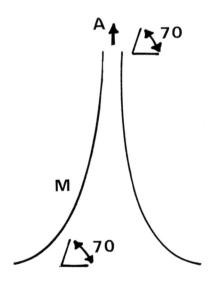

Fig. 11.8 Raubitscheck's parabolic astigmatic chart, typically printed black on a narrow white surround, the whole being on a medium grey background. The arrow shown at A can be printed to indicate a principal meridian. If the top parts of the two lines were equally clear, showing a 'best line' meridian, would the arrow indicate the required minus cylinder axis? Suppose only a part of one curve (near M) is clear. Since this part is oriented 70 degrees from the horizontal, which way would you rotate the arrow so that the clear part of the curve appears to move upwards? Would you move it the same way, whether the chart was being used 'direct' or as seen in a mirror?

minus cylindrical power is applied, progressive power extending the clarity along the limbs until the extremities are all clear.

Most astigmatic charts can be modified to good effect by providing black lines with high contrast by surrounding them with a white background; near this, surrounding the white and forming the main part of the background is a grey (approx. 50 per cent reflection factor). When blurred the black and white images merge into the grey.

Use lines of a suitable width for fans and blocks, 5 mm often being used for a chart viewed at 6 metres.

Mirror images of the scales should give no trouble to the optometrist, who usually faces in the opposite direction to that which confronts the patient. Some patients find this confusing and need help since they try to compensate for the mirror image. A question such as 'is it on your right?' just needs to be reinforced by a simultaneous gentle tap on the patient's right shoulder, without frightening the victim. This helps the optometrist to locate a line on the patient's right, say along 120 on the trial frame, which the optometrist may be viewing on the optometrist's left. (See Fig. 11.9.)

11.5   Tolerances in subjective refraction

However confident either patient or optometrist (or both) may be that a 'best' combination of lenses has been achieved, some doubt should persist. It *should* persist! The fact that those with low VA, even a few with good VA, tend not to notice small changes in lens power reminds us that there is a depth of focus for retinal images; this is related to depth of field in the photographic sense and to factors such as pupil size.

Adamson and Fincham (1939) described 'physiological ocular tolerance', the range of vergence within which there is no adjustment of accommodation; it is about 0.50, that is plus or minus 0.25D. Their 'perceptual tolerance' was understood to be based upon vision remaining clear despite a measured change of accommodation but it could refer to changes of vergence at the retina while accommodation is fixed. Refractive states of between about + 0.25D and – 0.25D were found to apply for distant objects, or about + 3.75D and + 4.50D for an object at 25 cm. Binocular and monocular amounts of these tolerances were not much different. It was suggested that binocular acceptance of more plus power could be evidence that binocular tolerance is greater than monocular in an individual. Reducing slight fogging could overestimate hyperopia by 0.50D.

Detection of the endpoint of clarity, when best VA is being sought, can differ in accuracy among patients. Layton *et al.* (1978) used binocular assessment of the earliest reporting of blur, when fogged 1.00D, as objects were moved further than one metre from the eyes. The data suggested that patients' VA can remain the same over a range of lens changes.

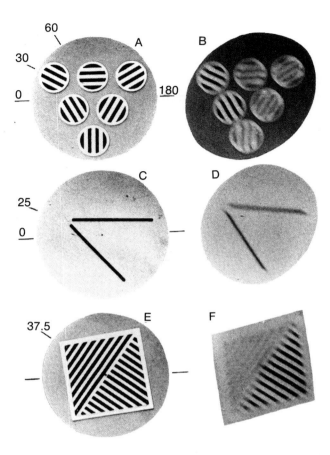

Fig. 11.9 A patient's view of astigmatic tests without a mirror.

The left column shows three 'direct' charts, presented at six metres to an astigmatic patient who views them through the 'best sphere'. The right column shows what the patient sees, by this direct view. Readers who usually use a mirror and reversed charts will have to think about the answers to this sequence.

A shows six 'blocks' set in 30 degree steps, like a fan chart. The patient reports a 'best line' between 30 and 60 degrees, relative to the trial frame protractor on the frame he is wearing. B shows his view. C shows a 'V' chart orientated along the meridian 25 degrees on the patient's frame, still viewed directly. D shows that the lower limb is reported as being the clearer. Which way should the point of the V then be rotated to equalize the limbs?

E shows two 'blocks' orientated to 37.5 degrees, which was the position at which the V limbs became equal. F shows the patient's view of the blocks in that orientation. What should the axis of the correcting minus cylinder be? The answer is not 37.5 degrees but the sum of 37.5 and 90 degrees.

Assuming that the patient could adequately identify the correct pair of blocks in chart A, which pair could you use instead of the V chart and which pair could you use instead of the chart in E?

Any consideration of the accuracy of patients' responses must be linked to the performance of the optometrist. The patient, through 'tolerances', fatigue, nervousness or a desire to say what is thought to be expected, can influence the subjective refraction and spasm of accommodation sometimes intrudes. Distraction or haste on the part of the optometrist or use of out-of-date data can be as unhelpful as bad questioning or unkind attitudes. Fatigue, even nervousness, can affect optometrists! Wray (1971) described several factors which undermine accuracy. If all clerical errors are avoided there are many snags to consider, such as the different forms of lenses, the manner in which an 'end point' is approached or the accuracy of axis directions on charts and trial frames. Vertex distances should be considered in all but low lens powers. The prescription for near tasks requires special thought. It is constructive to regard the subject accuracy of refraction with the crossed cylinder as ±0.25D in cyl power, or some 3 degrees in axis, somewhat depending on the power. Fan and block fogging methods probably have a similar accuracy of axis determination but rather better for power, even ±0.12D.

11.6   Binocular and balancing methods

Single binocular vision with foveal fusion is the usual, normal, situation. It may dictate modification to monocular prescriptions, given a chance, because of dominance of one eye, heterophoria, the demands of convergence or special work conditions. Ocular aberrations may be effectively altered by pupil variations, themselves influenced by convergence and accommodation. The effects of spherical aberration can be modified by the Stiles Crawford Effect I, while astigmatism may alter with pupil size.

Understandably, occlusion of one eye could make a patient feel that vision has been deprived of essential elements. While 'balancing' the VA of each eye as far as possible it is sometimes best to leave the dominant eye with the better VA. Rapidly alternating monocular occlusion is a quick but rough way to prompt the patient to express any noticeable difference between the two views; lens adjustments can remove the difference.

Prisms have been used to produce displaced images for comparison but a simple septum or polarization will usually be preferable. Most cases stand to gain from a binocular refinement of the prescription but is most helpful in aniso-metropes, amblyopes and those with questionable stability of binocular vision.

Image degradation

Foveal vision can be blurred or degraded monocularly or binocularly by fogging lenses or neutral density filters; peripheral vision remains. The prescription of each eye can then be optimized independently, under binocular conditions. Alternatively, some + 1.00DS to + 2.00DS may be added binocularly as fogging lenses, then reduced suitably with minus spheres until the two blurred percepts are equal. One eye at a time should subsequently have its fogging further reduced to find the best spherical and astigmatic corrections.

Polarizing

Crossed polarizing filters are built into some charts, permitting binocular fusion of parts of the fields of vision but with adequate monocular separation. Letters which are seen binocularly give a useful clue to the way any monocular modifications are accepted. Orientation of the planes of polarization obliquely along 45 and 135 degrees permits the 'visor' or clip holding the two analysers to be inverted (rather than cumbersome reversal R to L) to reverse the observation of letters or of stereo tests.

Many applications of the method reduce the effective chart luminance. The choice of the type of polarizing filter to give best 'cut out' is influenced by any residual colour and there is inevitably some absorption by filters. A dark element can obtrude when a 'contralateral' part of a chart is masked. Thus by careful design one may produce a very dark character (often rather gross) on a lighter background, or a light image on a very dark ground.

Grolman (1966) showed the advantages of 'vectograph' polarizing, using high resolution printing, high contrast and a bright binocular field.

Septum methods

Between 1936 and 1939 Turville introduced his 'infinity balance' technique, later adapted (with less success) for near vision. The early apparatus was an opaque rectangle fixed centrally to a mirror. Various modifications include erecting a vertical bar half way to a 'direct' chart or hanging a vertical white bar down the centre of a mirror. The bar is usally 30 mm wide. A rectangle 30 mm wide and 50 mm high permits a complete surrounding frame (such as a square) which is usually called a 'binocular lock'. Figures 11.10 and 11.11 indicate the principles.

Despite matching the luminance and colour of the septum to the chart there is a tendency for the septum to disturb some patients. They may converge and accommodate for it. Some astute developments by John Cole (1945) will now be rescued from the mists of antiquity. He used pairs of letters with TIB presentation, ranging from six-metre letters to 18-metre sizes. A 36-metre letter for one eye was

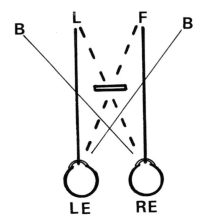

Fig. 11.10   A septum obscures the letter L from the RE and the letter F from the LE. Both eyes observe the 'binocular lock' BB. The septum is normally seen in physiological diplopia.

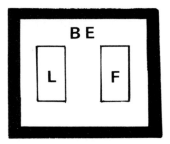

Fig. 11.11   The patient's view of the frame which acts as the 'binocular lock', the diplopic septum and the two monocular letters.

even paired with a spot light for a non-responsive eye, when necessary. Cole showed how monocular suppression can be found with one size but not with a larger letter. If ±0.25DS is added to the tentative prescription for one eye it can enhance single binocular vision.

Balancing

Using the septum or polarizing separation, first establish that each eye does see what it is intended to see. For example F for the RE and L for the LE. Fusion into 'E' can be prevented by prisms and many patients need a little base in prism.

If each eye sees as clearly as the other, apply + 0.25DS first to one eye then to the other, expecting to introduce the logical differences between the views of the monocular letters. Be prepared for 'acceptance' monocularly and even a favourable effect on binocular letters. If necessary resort to − 0.25DS (or more!) to achieve equality but if the extra power seems excessive suspect that something has happened of which you are unaware; possibly a cylinder has moved.

Initial inequality of visual acuity can be revealed, even a difference in colour of the images. Sometimes a discerning or fussy patient can be slightly disturbed (and demanding) as a result. Extra plus or minus for the less clear eye usually helps but you may be forced into a modification which reduces the better image somewhat, complete with explanations to the patient. Dominant eyes deserve consideration under such situations; some would also take into account 'handed-ness'. In some cases rapid X cyl adjustments can be very valuable.

11.7   Cycloplegic refraction

This approach tends to overcome difficulties caused by accommodation. It introduces factors likely to affect the eventual success of any prescription but the benefits usually outweigh these factors. Naturally the use of cycloplegia is chiefly for children and for younger adults.

A marked change in the attitudes to cycloplegics among North American optometrists has probably escaped the notice of younger UK colleagues. Forty years ago, legally denied the use of suitable drugs in practice, most North American optometrists expressed neither the need nor the desire for such help in some refractions. Alternative techniques were even vaunted as being superior. Since cycloplegia has become almost universally available to optometrists in the USA and newer cycloplegics have become acceptable alternatives to older ones such as atropine in so many cases, the situation has changed. Few optometrists can ignore the benefits, provided suitable selection of cases is made and appropriate precautions are applied. The possibility of an optometrist being accused of malpractice because cycloplegia was not used must be considered. Classé (1989) has shown how in the case of Kahn v. Shaw in 1941 an optometrist was actually pronounced 'negligent' in such a situation despite his not being permitted to use cycloplegia at the time. Considerations such as this need to be discussed with supervisors during the pre-registration year, since some of an older generation may have their own approach. At times the present writer's father, while proficient in cycloplegic techniques, preferred to refer certain patients rather than refract them under cycloplegia. While few today would endorse this excessive caution, there is no reason to go to such an extreme as to ignore the potential dangers.

It is necessary to take into account post-cycloplegic refraction data before prescribing. The careful screening of the eyes before using any cycloplegic or mydriatic is essential, with special care as to the state of the filtration angle and the retina.

The compensation for ciliary muscle tonus, usually one dioptre, made when atropine cycloplegia has been used, reduces most plus prescriptions. Relatively weak drugs such as cyclopentolate may need rather less allowance for the interference with tonus. Some care is needed to assess the depth of cycloplegia, using measurements of the near point of accommodation.

Dilated pupils introduce slight complications but axes of astigmatic corrections seem to suffer less change under these conditions than the cylinder power and spherical prescription.

Readers will probably be familiar with the more standard texts such as Vale and Cox (1985) or O'Connor Davies *et al.* (1989), on account of the use of such sources in undergraduate courses. There is some sense in comparing these views with more 'standard ophthalmological' accounts, such as can be found in *System of Ophthalmology* by Duke-Elder, noting how several of the more recent textbooks on 'clinical ophthalmology' and suchlike pay scant attention to refraction under cycloplegia. Yet studies such as one by Zetterström (1985) are to be considered. She compared the use of atropine (with its domestic difficulties) to a combination of 0.85 per cent cyclopentolate and 1.5 per cent phenylephrine; no significant differences were discovered in the series of young children with refractive error ranging from $-3.00D$ to $+7.00D$. There was a useful and short discussion of the subject by Mets (1988), reviewing the relevant literature, showing the limited conditions under which dangers exist and supporting the combination of cyclopentolate and phenylephrine. The production of optometrically based books such as that by Bartlett and Jaanus (1989) should be taken as an indication of some serious attention given to the subject and the fact that those concerned about the clinical ramifications of cycloplegia should consult these texts.

The difficulty of administering exact doses by eyedrops are well known and this should be borne in mind, with the variations in responses shown by different subjects, particularly by those with different pigmentation.

11.8   Some less conventional techniques

Most of these approaches come under the category of desperate measures so it is to be hoped that none shall be needed in the PQE; few examiners are likely to be impressed, on the assumption that cases of extraordinary difficulty are hardly likely to be used under such circumstances.

A personal experience may introduce the subject. Acting as a locum for a sick friend, delayed by fog on a long journey and arriving to find a packed waiting room plus a very strange refractor head was the natural opportunity. A somewhat difficult lady was completely unable to show agreement with my estimate of her RE axis of 20 for a cyl of 0.75D; rather she insisted, subjectively, that it should be 160! Considerable pressure, on account of wartime, prompted me to prescribe the relatively common flat form for her lenses, with PRO shape which was also the usual alternative to 'quadra', the new-fangled shape. Thus, at the crunch, when the spectacles were fitted, it was simple to try the new lens both ways and to substantiate the correct axis. Readers are at liberty to guess which it was.

Patients who do not respond to your 'normal' refractive procedures can be puzzling. Some need huge changes of power before they notice any difference, possibly because they have their own odd criteria. There are those who insist on commenting upon the colours being introduced as you change lenses, usually in connection with fan and block techniques; one way to remedy this difficulty is to add a yellow filter. Incidentally, the yellow filter does help some with low VA, especially for reading and there may be a temptation to use it when complaints flow about a fused bifocal for a myope.

Guided by objective methods, not just retinoscopy as the keratometer can help, you can usually coax some subjective approval of your efforts, The range of pinholes you so wisely possess will be useful; at least this gives hope that some improvement is possible. Guesswork can be reduced by the application of a 1.5 mm wide stenopaeic slit, slowly rotating this until the patient expresses more satisfaction, as each principal meridian is 'refracted' in turn. See Chapter 19, case 19.

Permitting the patient to rotate a cylinder herself rather suggests failure on the part of the refractionist but it often works wonders, even if it fails to flatter your skill. This happens mostly with fairly high astigmatic corrections. Sometimes the lenses in a trial frame move unhelpfully; possibly the patient shakes the head excessively. Some Plasticine or Blu-Tac can be helpful.

Oculo-rotatory reflexes, which shift the orientation of the eyes and therefore the axis of a required cylinder, have been used to check the axis position. With the tentative cylinder firmly in place in the trial frame, or in the refraction unit, produce carefully controlled tilts of the patient's head in opposite directions and to equal extents; the VA may be expected to be equally spoiled if the axis is correct, otherwise a better direction may be indicated.

Finally, something to test your appreciation of and even your understanding of your refractive techniques, strictly for the calm water enjoyed after passing the PQE. Molteno and Molteno (1977) produced a remarkable slide rule ostensibly to assist those driven to attempt prescribing spectacles in remote places far from expert practitioners. This copyright 'calculator' combines the conventional vision with near visual acuity obtained with a likely age-related addition, by asking the patient monocularly to thread a needle, first with red, then with green thread. This unconventional approach leads to adjustment of the circular slide rule and hopeful estimates of the best distance sphere, to be checked with a bichromatic test. An attempt to prescribe even cylinders is included.

The 'Optomat' was obtainable via Box 5454, Dunedin, New Zealand, for those intrigued.

Chapter 12
The Near-vision Prescription

Many features of near vision as a visual task must be taken into account when prescribing. Available accommodation, the distances and sizes of all the stimuli involved, the luminances and contrasts, glare, the time permitted for short periods of viewing and the durations of working periods are other factors. Sometimes the health or medication of a patient is relevant. The influence of the degree of attention in use will emerge in section 12.2. Previous spectacle prescriptions and dispensing are important since the types and even the positions of lenses can have different effects. Contact lenses present some special aspects when used for near vision.

One of the most helpful rules to adopt, which is seldom to be disobeyed, is caution in making gross changes; often a change of no more than 0.75D is advisable. Unfortunately previous 'corrections' may not have been prescribed, but a relative's spectacles may have been adopted! At this stage the reader should find it useful to refer to some of the cases presented in Chapter 16.

12.1   Accommodation

The classical tables of amplitude of accommodation have stood the test of time fairly well. Although climatic and racial features tend to affect accommodation, the ways in which these sometimes appear to influence reading additions may chiefly be the result of prescribing habits. At any age expect a variation of about ±1.00D from the mean value in a population; the important need is for an individual's monocular amplitudes to be known since a difference of more than 0.50D can indicate the need for further investigation.

The depth of field at a typical reading distance of some 38 cm is greater with small pupils and may be reduced by unusually good visual acuity. Possibly readers may find some difficulty in reconciling the two statements just made; they could stimulate some practical experiments. In addition, the errors made in measuring amplitude of accommodation can be ±1.00D.

Much of what passes for accommodation really amounts to depth of field, particularly in presbyopes, as Wagstaff (1966) showed from objective tests.

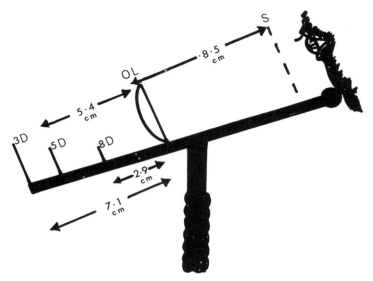

Fig. 12.1 Simple (Badel) Optometer for accommodation measurement. The angled bar is held against the patient's cheek so that a plus 10DS lens is approx. 10 cm from the eye, 8.5 cm from the spectacle plane. Small objects are fixed at suitable distances from the other side of the lens so that they require different amounts of accommodation referred to the spectacle plane. In the figure three distances are chosen for values of spectacle accommodation 3, 5 and 8 dioptres. The 5D value is suitable for ensuring that a tentative reading addition is likely to be adequate for normal distances between 33 and 40 cm.

There is some influence from the direction of the line of sight, often because the amount of support for the crystalline lens varies. The near point rule should be depressed to imitate the normal direction of gaze, using a mean of three readings. Simple Badel optometers can be handy for monocular measurements of accommodation referred to the spectacle plane (see Fig. 12.1). Association between accommodation and the innervation of convergence, as well as pupil size, must be considered when heterophoria is involved.

Accommodative failure, other than presbyopia

When protracted, this is termed 'insufficiency' of accommodation and the range and amplitude are both lower than expected for the patient's age. If merely a temporary, slight, difficulty it is usual to refer to 'ill sustained' accommodation. Sometimes it is possible to detect an excessive reaction time, in 'inertia' of accommodation. Before considering a spectacle prescription as more than a temporary measure the cause must be discovered. Some pathological process, general bodily disease, severe sinus or dental conditions, alcohol poisoning,

Graves' disease or even hysteria may be among the possibilities. Ocular conditions such as glaucoma or intra-ocular infection (particularly cyclitis) may be involved.

Complete paralysis of accommodation, a very serious matter, may be caused from systemic drugs, various diseases or traumas and may be monocular or binocular. It is important to investigate associated pupil anomalies.

After the cause has been treated it is usual to prescribe plus spheres, possibly with prism assistance and to maintain a regular watch on the situation. In some cases accommodative exercises are used, notably binocular reading at different distances.

In some work situations, such as mining or in military activity at night, low luminances can lower the accommodative responses, when high spatial frequency information is not assimilated, but most difficulty tends to be with objects nearer than 66 cm. Those with low visual acuity may suffer in the same way, thus requiring more plus than might be expected.

Protracted spells of very intense close work, such as VDU viewing have been shown to result in a temporary lowering of accommodative response.

Accommodative spasm, or excessive ciliary tonus

Several types exist, manifested as a pseudo-myopia giving blurred distance vision, headaches and possibly macropsia. Various drugs or irritation of the para-sympathetic system can be involved so the patient may not always be the adolescent 'crammer' or pre-presbyope more naturally considered to be liable to these symptoms. Ocular or brain stem inflammation must be ruled out, also some form of hysteria. If there is a recent history of trauma that may be important. Having taken care of possible sinister causes, for example through the GP, it is usual to involve a cycloplegic refraction than to prescribe suitable plus for as long as really necessary; orthoptic assistance may be used, even hypnosis in some cases. Recent suggestions that 'biofeedback' training can assist these cases must be noted, with caution, and those interested would find comments and references given by Reeves (1989) among the most helpful.

The 'Mandelbaum effect' and various forms of 'night myopia', mostly associated with tonic accommodation and an involuntary accommodative effort, can be considered here. People who work behind a close screen, such as ticket office clerks, may succumb to the stimulus provided by the screen; they tend habitually to over-accommodate. Driving at night or in a featureless fog, similarly induces a 'rest' position of accommodation, which is between one and two dioptres.

Short accounts of accommodative mechanisms can be found in Fletcher (1954a), Cooper (1987) and Stark (1988).

12.2   Dynamic retinoscopy ('DR')

Do not confuse this retinoscopy with near fixation, usually at 66 cm, where relaxation of accommodation is encouraged when seeking a distance prescription. Dynamic retinoscopy was used in various ways, encouraging convergence and accommodation for targets some 33 cm from the spectacle plane, many years before extensive British interest between 1930 and 1950. A reconciliation between differing views of L.A. Swann and S. Taylor can be read in the account by Taylor (1939) and the closing stages of much interesting correspondence are in the *Optician* newspaper up to May 1947.

Some optometrists greatly value the procedure. It is surprising that many others do not use it, particularly as it has been claimed to speed up arrival at a prescription. This summary presents basic aspects, encouraging you to make some personal trials. In the PQE, however, caution may incline you sensibly to avoid the technique, in case any discussion with the examiner tends, shall we say, to become unproductive.

A major difficulty can be the apparatus. Some retinoscopes provide an illuminated 'mini-chart' a little in front of and below the sight hole, and an externally illuminated substitute can be attached. It must carry a few small letters and a ring of tiny dots, perhaps with a couple of larger dots among these. The orange filter recommended in section 10.1 will be particularly welcome to the patient here, to reduce the glare from the retinoscope beam. A similar target can be mounted on a pencil so that you can move it towards the patient, keeping the retinoscope at the original 33 cm. Drive the retinoscope beam horizontally across the two eyes, and note any differences between the two. It will be surprising if you do not notice the reduction of the appearance of spherical aberration in the retinoscope reflex, since lens changes and miosis combine to this end.

Binocular spherical additions, increasing in power from + 0.50DS to + 2.50DS, for both eyes, are almost essential equipment. Today such 'dynamic racks' of pairs of lenses are not readily available but two single retinoscopy racks (see Figs. 12.2 and 12.3) can be locked together. Steps of 0.25DS are ideal but 0.50DS steps could be tried. The lenses slide up and down either side of the nose so small lenses no larger than 30 mm diameter or square lenses are needed. Centres are usually 60 mm apart. A plastics mount, with a handle at one side is not too difficult to have made. Coated lenses would be ideal. Some refraction units are difficult to advance binocularly, without an assistant.

Monocular DR

This has a limited use, for example as an objective check on accommodation or to help a decision on a medium-to-high cylinder power or axis for near vision. Binocular axis changes from monocular axes are not unknown.

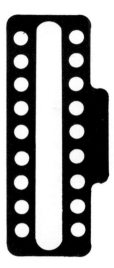

Fig. 12.2   A typical binocular rack of plus spheres for dynamic retinoscopy. Maximum space must be allowed for the nose, although the rack is likely to be held at an exaggerated vertex distance.

Convergence and accommodation

Notice the order of the words in this subheading. Convergence is normally the main binocular near-vision requirement and brings with it convergence-induced accommodation. Despite the glare with DR, good foveal fusion is likely; certainly when the patient is merely told to 'look at' the target, a peripheral fusion should exist. It is when critical attention is in action that precise convergence and relatively exact accommodation are exerted. The differences between these two types of near vision have caused most of the misunderstanding of DR.

With casual binocular vision the retinoscope shows an initial 'with' movement, capable of neutralization by increasing binocular plus spheres. We are assuming that a correct distance prescription is being worn; presbyopes should be wearing a tentative near correction. The 'with' movement can also disappear if the (fused) target is advanced towards the patient and eventually an 'against' reflex may emerge. This neutralization point, where 'with' just disappears, is the 'low neutral'. It can be seen in monocular vision as well and since lenses of about + 0.50DS or + 0.75DS usually produce it, there is some basis for attributing it to 'lag' of accommodation. It has been called the 'objective' lag but it is unlikely to be related to the plane of reflection where the vitreous and retina touch.

Critical binocular near vision

Near fixation with encouragement by the optometrist to count the small dots, to note how many are larger than most, etc., imitates the most realistic approach.

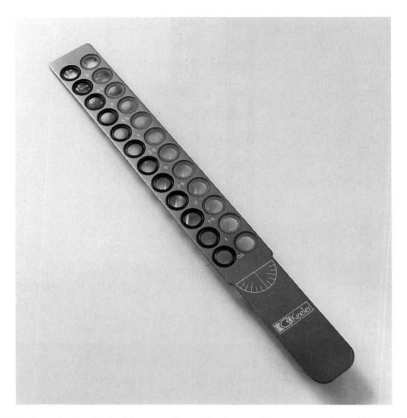

Fig. 12.3 A rack of spherical lenses, plus and minus, often a convenient aid for retinoscopy. (Courtesy of Keeler Ltd.)

Reflex accommodation induced by convergence amounts to about 1 dioptre per metre angle of convergence up to 30 years, with a drop to about 0.25D by age 50. Critical vision augments this stimulus. Other factors such as heterophoria and presbyopia obviously intrude so that excessive innervation to counteract exophoria is likely to induce more accommodation, when less plus is needed to reach 'neutral' with the retinoscope. If the patient fails to converge at any moment the reflex can be seen to alter. A little experimenting with base in and base out prisms is instructive.

Removal of 'with' movement is likely to persist as extra plus is added, beyond the 'low neutral', presumably because a form of 'negative relative accommodation' (virtually a relaxation of accommodation) takes place. A 'high neutral' is reached, after which the addition of extra plus sphere makes the reflex 'against'. It is usually necessary to encourage critical vision to obtain this and a value of + 1.50DS is expected up to age 30. In casual binocular near vision the plus required to obtain neutral may be more than the usual value; switching to critical vision and inducing extra accommodation can change the 'neutral' to 'against'.

Presbyopes should be wearing a tentative near vision prescription and the 'high neutral' value is sought in addition to any reading addition incorporated. Early presbyopes probably require for reading about 0.50DS less plus than the 'high neutral', while over 60 years the 'high neutral' is more often produced by the likely addition required.

It is important to develop a personal method which suits your techniques, interpreting the data in the light of near prescriptions proven by other methods before placing too much reliance on your DR results.

Undoubtedly 'accommodative lag' is partly a manifestation of an optical system not strictly in focus, capable of tolerating some blur subjectively and being content with less than maximum effort. Some teachers might accept a comparison with students! Also, vice versa!

Objective balancing of near-vision prescriptions is readily performed with DR and since this can be done without a binocular rack of lenses it is an excellent starting exercise.

Accommodation

Although 'lag' and relaxation of accommodation can be approached along the lines proposed it is more difficult to assess amplitude of (positive) accommodation. Taking each eye in turn under similar conditions you can obtain an idea as to inequality of amplitudes of accommodation.

Retinoscopy through minus lenses in the young requires a mobile target of high interest value, moved in from the retinoscope. Older patients more sedately build up 'against' reflex movement, until giving up the effort.

Prescribing from DR

Remember that the correct distant spectacle correction should be in place in a young patient and the tentative near prescription in a presbyope. Reassessment of the near vision situation, particularly spherical balance, can then involve DR. Exceptionally, DR is the initial approach, superseding distance fixation retinoscopy or subjective methods. This may be for a handicapped patient who presents special difficulty. A few optometrists have used DR initially as a routine, as a personal foible. Most would feel more secure having reconfirmed reversal with distance fixation.

Prism modifications can be used to manipulate the neutral positions but the information must take its place among other data, including subjective factors, as in all prescribing.

12.3   Astigmatic corrections in near vision

It is about one hundred years since suggestions of 'astigmatic accommodation' (deliberate or involuntary reduction of astigmatism by unequal contractions of the ciliary muscle) arose. The reasons why the present writer prefers to use the term 'astigmatism accidentally introduced during accommodation' are explained at length by Fletcher (1951–52; 1954b) Briefly, many conditions can be mistaken for astigmatic accommodation, there being a well known optical phenomenon which makes near vision spectacle astigmatism slightly greater than the distance correction, provided accommodation is used. Figures 12.4 and 12.5 give some examples in which the influence of distance spherical corrections is shown as well as the importance of accommodation. The vertex distance is involved and a useful approximation by Swaine (see FLetcher 1954b) includes the distance sphere, S, the assumed accommodative effort, A, and the vertex distance in metres, d.

Thus:

$$\frac{\text{Near vision cylinder}}{\text{Distance vision cylinder}} = (1 + \frac{dA}{1 - ds})^2$$

It is obvious that theoretically these modifications are significant only to high power astigmatic corrections. A few per cent increase is to be expected.

More important in practice are the cases where changes in astigmatic correction are required because of 'accidental' changes, presumably caused by asymmetries in the crystalline lens, zonule or ciliary body. It is unlikely that these cases will be found unless retinoscopy or cross cylinder refraction is carried out with accommodation operating. This is unlikely, as a routine, therefore it is usually when patients complain of near vision difficulty with 'correct' prescriptions that the changes needed are discovered. Naturally, these may not depend on the strength of the distance astigmatism. Fig. 12.6 shows how the theoretical increase of some 0.37DC was insufficient in one young patient, who required twice that difference in power for near vision. Rapid use of crossed cylinders, using a near vision chart monocularly and concentrating on the clarity of round letters, is helpful whenever such situations are suspected.

12.4   Near-vision additions

Rare cases of accommodative paresis in the young are in need of extra plus power for close work but most 'additions' are for presbyopes. No wonder that the SMC adopted the motto 'A blessing to the aged'. Causes of presbyopia may include the changes in the ciliary body, such as a weakening of the muscular force from intrusion of connective tissue, the increase in shape of the region and possible differences in innervation. However, Stark (1988) and Weale (1989) describe factors such as changes in the crystalline lens as being most important. It appears

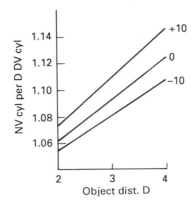

Fig. 12.4 Effects of object distance (in the presence of accommodation) and of distance spherical prescription (– 10 to + 10DS) on the factor by which distant vision cylinder must be multiplied to give theoretical near vision cylinder, for a vertex distance of 15 mm. (See Fletcher 1952 & 1954.)

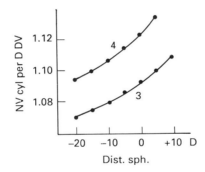

Fig. 12.5 Effects of distance spherical prescription and of two values of nomimal accommodation (3 and 4D) on the factor by which distant vision cylinder must be multiplied to give theoretical near vision cylinder, for a vertex distance of 15 mm. (Swaine's data, see Fletcher 1954.)

that convergence associated with accommodation is affected by age less than accommodation itself, while convergence induced accommodation is reduced in older people.

The manifestations of presbyopia are well known as difficulty with near vision, a tendency to hold books at arm's length, asthenopia and a need for more light on the task. It is usually considered that about one-third of the accommodative amplitude should be maintained as a 'reserve' during sustained near vision and this is often a basis for prescribing. A method of arriving at the near addition gives approximately the same average additions as the one-third in reserve approach. Thus at age 45 'acceptable' additions ranged from zero to + 1.00DS, mean

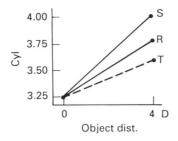

Fig. 12.6 Astigmatic changes in one eye of a young subject normally corrected by − 2.00/ − 3.25 × 180. The theoretical change for a vertex distance of 15 mm is shown (T) for 4D nominal accommodation. The retinoscopic increase of 0.50DC is shown for fixation at ¼ metre as (R) and the subjective (crossed cyl) change of 0.75DC is shown as (S). (See Fletcher 1954.)

0.50DS; at 50 the lowest addition was 0.50DS, the highest was + 2.00DS and the mean was + 1.25DS, while the comparable figures at age 60 were + 1.25DS + 2.5ODS and + 2.00DS.

Millodot and Millodot (1989) discussed the 'one-third in reserve rule' and made comparisons with the 'one-half reserve' alternative, which they found better suited to women over 52 and men over 63.

Above all, treat each patient as an individual, ensuring that all real needs are discussed and that no excessive additions are prescribed. Explain with care, if possible reinforcing this with a booklet, that there is likely to be a reduced depth of field, a reduced working distance and distance or intermediate blur.

A detailed consideration of the effective powers of trial and prescription lenses in near vision by Rabbetts and Bennett (1986) showed that when the near addition was made with the extra lens in front of the distance correction in a trial frame small differences were found with two different forms of trial lens. Only with distance powers over + 10DS were there significant variations. Some advantages were noted when plano surfaces of reduced aperture trial lenses were nearer the eye. The differences produced by refraction units can be determined only if the internal optical characteristics of individual instruments are known, so do not overlook the possibility of difficulties of this type.

Intermediate prescriptions, with appropriate 'additions' for music, library shelves, cash registers or VDU terminals must not be overlooked. Positions and distances, plus all other relevant factors, must be taken into account. Horgen *et al.* (1989) have demonstrated how correction of presbyopia by different forms of lenses, can influence work posture and muscle loads in the back and shoulder region. In many cases a single vision lens was preferable to multi-focal or progressive forms.

Despite or, perhaps, because of the reappearance of 'ready-made' spectacles (self prescribed) in the UK it is important to stress the need for near-vision prescriptions to be dispensed with care. Attention to prismatic effects, to unequal additions which may be required, and to differences in the heights of the two eyes are among the necessary steps to success. The angles of lenses relative to the visual axes are important, assuming that the optical axis should coincide with the line of sight in most cases.

Chapter 13
Changes in Refractive Errors

Much statistical data is available about how refractive errors are produced, the different possibilities for the relationships between the ocular structures and their powers and how development is likely to take place. Individuals are likely to be ignored since they are used to build up the statistics, although in a clinical situation a patient may be regarded as falling into one of the many 'categories'. Thus we may look at one myope as 'axial', possibly because of the fundus features and the fairly flat cornea.

Several phases are distinguishable, as most individuals become older. There is a batch of possibilities for premature babies, we have certain expectations for a normal Scandinavian neonate, 'critical' periods are understood to emerge early in development, growth towards and after puberty is recognized while landmarks and trends appear in adults and 'the aged'. With experience, optometrists discover much of this for themselves and begin to relate likely changes in refractive error to stages of life.

Minimal study of these matters needs to be selective, for example by noting how Olson (1987) explained the needs of visually impaired children and sampling parts of the lengthy and well-documented review Borish (1970) or the concise text on ageing of the eye by Weale (1963).

13.1 Assorted changes

Genetic and environmental factors affect most of the changes in the eyes of an individual. At the chairside the optometrist is concerned with the means and percentiles of textbooks less than with the immediate situation of the patient. Parents understandably often seek an opinion as to causes and prognosis of a child's ametropia. At all ages, in most cases, there are questions (expressed or mute) such as 'what produced this refractive state, what does it mean today and how might it change?' Such interest does not only apply to the 'progressive' myope, to the aphakic infant, to the diabetic or to incipient keratoconus; most patients deserve consideration along these lines, with suitable comment. At the

116

present time 'radial keratotomy' has added to the questions, as shown in the Prospective Evaluation of Radial Keratotomy (PERK) Study and described, for instance, by Bourque *et al.* (1986).

This text must confine itself chiefly to the more mundane changes and rather briefly. Certainly it must stimulate an awareness of certain usual expectations.

One group of changes, not particularly related to ageing, revolves around relatively sinister ocular situations. While it is known that upper lid pressure from extended reading periods or from meibomian cysts (see Chapter 19, cases 17 and 32) may distort corneas and alter refraction temporarily, there are worse possibilities.

Pathological changes in the cornea, surgery on the eye, chemical insult or malnutrition can affect vision, sometimes by altering the spectacle prescription. Retinal tumours and centroserous chorioretinopathy tend to produce relative hyperopia; in the latter condition there are often seasonal variations, more young males are involved, and several additional warning signs, but the refractive error can alert you to the situation. Diabetic eyes (if phakic) suffer variations in lenticular power which include transient myopia during hyperglycaemic phases. Drugs such as miotics or sulphonamides, or toxic conditions can alter refraction. An important point is that 'unexpected' changes in ocular refraction raise suspicions. Hence, what is to be 'expected'?

13.2   Trends in youth

European babies are normally moderately hyperopic at first, with some exceptions, therefore their visual needs and their accommodation are linked with their binocular status. Very early determination of the neonatal child's situation usually holds the key to development. As Banks (1980) and others have shown, astigmatic errors of significance in full-term babies are few but tend to become more prevalent in the first few months, only to decrease in frequency by the average age of a year. During the second year astigmats become slightly fewer. Naturally the difficulties and likely methods of arriving at these refractive errors make the findings somewhat unreliable.

In Fig. 13.1 what should be the familiar tendency to change in 'mean' equivalent spherical ametropia has been simplified. From the infant hyperopia, happily catered for in most cases by accommodation, a more myopic distance refraction emerges around puberty or, as some might prefer, as school work becomes more serious. True, sometimes this change is expressed as either an early or a late 'myopic development' and in certain cultures environmental factors or changes in work habits can become involved. Fig. 13.2 demonstrates something of the trend seen in Fig. 13.1. Here an individual female patient's right eye prescription has been plotted over three decades, starting with cycloplegic

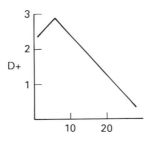

Fig. 13.1 Early trends in European refractive errors. The relative increase in hyperopia manifested before nine years moves into the myopic trend in a typical schoolchild.

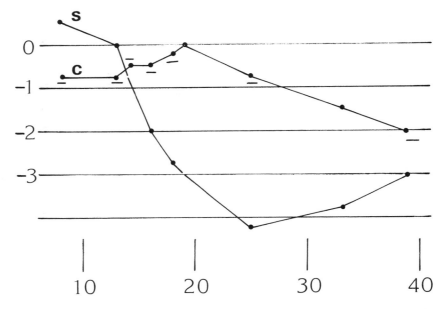

Fig. 13.2 Thirty years of refractive changes. The woman was virtually emmetropic to the mid-teens, after which a strong progression of myopia emerged, without fundus changes. Paternal grandmother highly myopic (some 25D) and several brothers and sisters of mother are moderate myopes.

refraction. A need for a myopic correction was discovered during teenage driving lessons, when it was clear that she might fail the test of reading car number plates.

One expects about 0.50D of with the rule astigmatism in youth, tending to against the rule with increasing years; here the cyl axis remained almost constantly horizontal, while the amount rose between 20 and 40 years. Note the change in spherical power after age 25. By contrast, the right eye data over twenty years of another patient's life, shown in Fig. 13.3 show atypical alterations. There is an

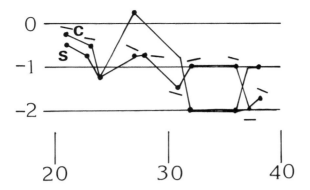

Fig. 13.3 Two decades in a man's refractive history. The eye experienced progression of an inherited lens condition. (See Fig. 13.4.)

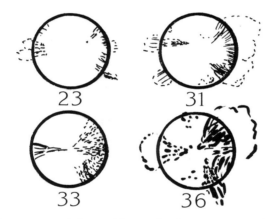

Fig. 13.4 Lens changes recorded over 13 years in the same eye as shown in Fig. 13.3.

inherited lenticular condition underlying the variations and Fig. 13.4 represents sketches made at intervals from age 23 to age 36.

13.3 Trends in later years

In Fig. 13.5 another rise in relative hyperopia can be seen in averaged data for spherical equivalent ametropias, between 40 and 70 years of age. This is usually described as a 'senile' hyperopia, expected to be accompanied by a move towards against-the-rule astigmatism of some half a dioptre, or changes in these directions from a refractive error well removed from the mean value in a given population. After 70 comes the senile myopic trend and various explanations have been suggested for these variations.

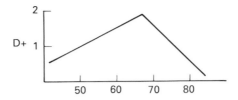

Fig. 13.5 Adulthood and typical refractive changes in spherical ametropia.

Fig. 13.6 gives an example, a lady patient seen over the years between ages 45 and 65. The spherical trend is largely as anticipated. The astigmatism stayed remarkably stable, with slight swings of axis which were undeniably preferred by this very discerning (not fussy) patient. At the same time the figure shows the increase in reading addition. Note the last slight reduction in addition, as the hyperopia reached + 1.50DS, which was at the same time as the patient was prescribed a + 1.00DS addition for intermediate distance viewing of a wordprocessor. Many years before, at about 53 years of age, she was provided with a weak plus in lorgnette form for shopping and looking at notes when addressing meetings.

The change in astigmatism most likely to have taken place is seen to a limited extent in Fig. 13.7 which represents the refractive errors of a male patient who has been under the care of the author over some 30 years. The data again relates to only one eye, in fact one in which the VA has remained at about 6/5 throughout, with very little change in the crystalline lens. A healthy, vigorous individual, this man shows no sign of the myopic dip of the graph which might be expected.

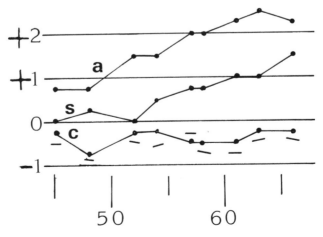

Fig. 13.6 Refractive errors and presbyopic additions in a woman from 45 to 66 years of age. Note the similarity between the spherical error and Fig. 13.5.

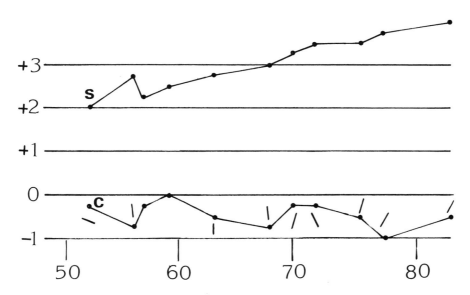

Fig. 13.7 Refractive changes in a man over three decades. Presbyopic additions are not shown but they were typical.

It is seldom that the expected trend is the only way that a prescription can be modified but in the author's experience it has been necessary at times to send replacement spectacles to patients 'marooned' in distant lands and unable to secure any other replacement; in such cases the slight modification 'prescribed' on the basis of experience has invariably been acceptable, probably as the result of 'Hobson's choice'. Such remote control of a situation is only an extreme last resort. Reviews of the changes in adulthood which are worth reading are by Morgan (1960) and Hirsch (1960).

Chapter 14
Aspects of Prescribing

Serious students of optometry and discerning patients who have benefited from extensive service from the profession recognise the complex nature of many of the decisions involved. There is a somewhat daunting responsibility facing the novice optometrist, hence the extensive education and the present examinations required after graduation. Time and study must be added to achieve increasing competence.

Extraordinary ideas are emerging at the time of writing, tending to some regression in the quality of eye care in the UK. The encouragement of self-choice spectacles and the reduction of some aspects of eye examination are such proposals. Since public experience has chiefly led to progress in optometry, eventually time must reverse this deleterious trend and overmuch reliance on automated procedures such as computerized refraction devices used without discernment. Optometrists will continue to gain data from a variety of new instruments but the personal element will remain paramount. As in other branches of health care, in much advice about finance, with legal guidance or even ways partners in marriage are found, there is a limit to the service provided by machines.

14.1 Responsible prescribing

Patients arrive with real or potential needs, requiring eye examination, the determination of ametropia and investigation of binocular vision. At the stage of prescribing 'optical appliances' dispensing must be under consideration, unless advice is that no 'prescription' is required. Having assembled the data the optometrist assesses the situation, with suitable discussion with the patient or a child's parents and makes a decision. Experience and skill are involved, taking account of costs, the patient's wishes, even future travel or the prognosis of a disease. An important feature is sometimes the significance to the individual of a small change in prescription or the likely need for a first correction of minimal strength. The possible accusation of 'unnecessary prescribing' must be faced. Explanations are usually given to the patient. Decisions should be firm, positive and reasonably directive, although in a few cases it is essential to regard a prescription as an experiment, with early reassessment; steps of partial correction can lead to eventual acceptance of an optimum prescription. At times trial lenses must be used to show the potential of a fresh prescription, how picture frames or table tops will look, the view across the street or the difficulty of moving amid furniture or down stairs. Clip-on lenses or adhesive prisms are often helpful for such trials. Chapters 15 and 19 will expand on details of this theme. Note, for instance, cases 15 and 16 as well as cases 22 and 29.

A judgement as to how effective a small change of power could be must be based on all the information about the patient gathered during the whole eye examination and the refractive procedures. In section 11.5 the questions of tolerances and accuracy arose. Ignoring changes of 0.12D and the frequent habit of omitting very small astigmatic corrections in some reading corrections, there may be doubt as to the need for, say, a correction of $-0.25DC$ axis 45. One phlegmatic patient may be an obvious candidate for ignoring the cylinder. Another asthenopic and discerning patient could well benefit; yet supposing 'tolerance and accuracy' to suggest that either zero power or $-0.50DC$ axis 45 might be acceptable most prescribers would sensibly opt for the middle of that range. How the patient reacted previously would be valuable information.

14.2   Discovering the patient's needs

Without adequate questioning and sometimes some demonstration, it is all too easy to make wrong assumptions and to prescribe badly. In my first week of practice alone I overplussed a bank manager for desk work! It is useful to have available a collection of likely 'tasks' such as needles and cotton, lines of stitching, sheets of music, a steel rule, a keyboard and a TV screen, playing cards and a few nuts and bolts. With these, 'real' situations are rapidly imitated to assist the final prescription. In Italy, at least, a spectacle prescription includes the distance PD but sometimes the lens powers should be followed by a proposal for lens materials or forms, absorptive properties, etc.

An extensive consideration of 'visual task analysis' can be found in a previous text (Fletcher 1961) in a more industrial context. The main elements must suffice here, as follows. Several apply to every patient.

Angular sizes of detail to be discerned

Usually the visual acuity provided must meet the requirements, such as the size of a needle eye. When the gap is 0.01 cm and the nearness is 3D, using sensible units which are readily related to optometric affairs, the angular subtense is (0.01×3) = approx 0.1 prism dioptres. This should correspond to about 3 minutes of arc or a third of 'standard' visual acuity, not much different from 'N8' in near chart terms. It remains to be decided if the gap is the critical size, since it may be reduced in practice as the tip of thread obscures it. (See Fig. 14.1).

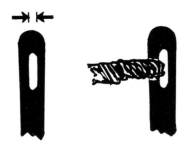

Fig. 14.1 Threading a needle as a 'visual task'. The critical gap, usually the width of the eye of the needle, requires moderate visual acuity if it is assumed that an average size eye is viewed alone. It is likely that at the moment of truth the detail is reduced in size as thread partially obscures the gap.

Contrasts of colour and brightness

Short of a demonstration or even a visit to a workplace, this feature is difficult to assess. Some patients will define the situation well and it is possible to make some measurements. A series of ten graded neutral papers is helpful, each with a small hole punched in it so that parts of the task can be matched for luminance. You can easily estimate the contrast of your test chart in this way. Munsell papers, paint manufacturers' samples or stamp collection gradings will do.

Luminance, a combination of reflectance and illuminance

The description of lamps according to wattage and distances is often only a start in assessing this important aspect. Shades, directions, glare and even colours are involved. A security guard patrolling under some sodium lighting while wearing Crookes lenses is at a peculiar disadvantage! When measurements of illuminance are possible it is helpful to have a small light meter, or at least a photographic exposure meter for which a simple conversion table for illuminance is easily produced.

Time and motion

Many occupations and a few home situations involve some limitations on visibility since only short periods of observation are possible. When it is difficult to advise extension of time, helpful attention may be given to extra illumination or the avoidance of stroboscopic effects. Attention to rest periods is a recognized method of relieving stress.

Hazards, at work, at play or in the home

Protection is sometimes as much a part of a prescription as correction.

Task format and familiarity

The style of a display, or printed material, often influences visibility, just as the positions involved may introduce difficulty.

14.3   Powers to prescribe

Students tend to be encouraged to obtain 'maximum plus' throughout their practice in refractive techniques, which amounts to minimum minus sphere in myopia. It is somewhat paradoxical that this attitude, sensibly aimed at avoiding excesses of accommodation, must be modified at the times when many prescriptions are written. Considering the usual six metres distance for optotypes as encouraging about 0.25D of accommodation for those who have enough and taking into account any 'night myopia' which may be induced by a dimly-lit room, some adjustment to the spherical power is possible; the conditions under which the prescription is to be used, heterophoria and other binocular matters and, of course, what was previously prescribed must be considered. Some of the effects of lenses will be covered in the next three sub-sections. The important attitude is to regard the data obtained during objective and subjective refraction as an extended base from which to arrive at the final powers.

The oft-repeated dictum that changes in power should seldom be greater than 0.75D should be applied to spherical and cylindrical prescriptions. Astigmatic corrections are frequently omitted when they are under 0.25D, particularly when the spherical elements of the prescription are likely to assist the relief of symptoms. Changes of cylinder power must be related to the 'equivalent' sphere, so that supposing a – 2.75DC is modified to – 1.25DC, extra minus sphere is indicated; whether this should be exactly half the 'drop' in cyl power is a matter to decide in company with the other final adjustments of spherical power, so either – 0.75DS or – 0.50DS might be ordered with the lower cylinder.

Changes in power are more tolerable when axes are not oblique. Axis modifications are wise if the change is potentially large. Relatively large alterations of axis, such as 30 degrees can be tolerated more readily for cylinders under 1.00D and it is easy to disturb the patient by altering a 3.00D cylinder more than a few degrees.

Very high myopias, which almost invariably have shown progression long after puberty, often demonstrate the degenerative axial elongation of the globe in various ways. There is likely to be peripapillary atrophy, large conus, staphyloma, choroidal atrophy and lenticular opacities. Associated abnormalities such as dystrophies are expected. Most of these 'pathological' myopias are accompanied by vitreous liquefaction and degeneration of both the peripheral and macular regions. The dangers of retinal detachment prompt referral for ophthalmological opinion; ERG records often show reduction from normality as one indication of the degeneration. A useful discussion of such myopias is by Goss and Eskridge (1987). It is rare to find a modern ophthalmological text which suggests conservative 'treatment' in such cases and when the decision is made to prescribe lenses it is usual to maximize the visual acuity; sometimes this involves magnification, where the VA is low.

Finally, a prescription should be issued with explanations. Every patient should be adequately informed about the state of the eyes, about the implications of any binocular disorder and possible distortions or other difficulties which the new lenses might induce.

14.4   Anisometropia and anisophoria

Where the powers for the two eyes are significantly different both prescribing and dispensing should be harmonized. Some factors tend to be antagonistic to each other, perhaps if binocular vision has to be enhanced by both equality of retinal images and by minimal prismatic variations. Anisophoria of the 'optical' type differentiated by Remole (1989) in a very useful exposition is concerned most with variations in prismatic deviation away from the optical centres of lenses, these lenses being well 'centred' for one direction of gaze. Lucid explanations have been given by Bennett (1971) in a review of optical centration of invisible bifocals and by Bennett and Rabbetts (1984a), which are excellent for revision.

There is considerable tolerance for variations of horizontal prism power but vertical discrepancies can be objectionable if over one prism dioptre. The adaptations which are possible have been investigated by North and Henson (1985); individual patients can demonstrate their own extent of acceptance of prism without diplopia or asthenopia. In anisometropia adaptations are often aided by the fact that the condition develops slowly; an exception would be unilateral aphakia. Careful assessment, well chosen questions and the trial of some alternative powers and prisms, using different head and eye positions, is a valuable guide. Fig. 14.2 shows a device specially constructed for one myopic anisometrope who was a candidate for a bifocal for office work; there was little chance of single binocular vision here, as with some anisometropes with large differences. An experiment such as this, using parts of simple plastics lenses, can often lead to a useful decision. Prism controlled bifocals are expensive but can meet the needs of presbyopes or anisometropes with adequate accommodation. Alternatively two pairs of spectacles, appropriately centred, can be used and it is part of the prescriber's function to be concerned with the way in which prescriptions can be dispensed.

A simple measurement of anisophoria is possible with an ordinary Maddox rod and a point source, used at suitable distances and held in different positions relative to the primary position of fixation.

14.5   Aniseikonia

It is strange, in view of the derivation, that this word is not spelt 'anisoeikonia', but the form used in the heading is now well entrenched. The causes of the unequal

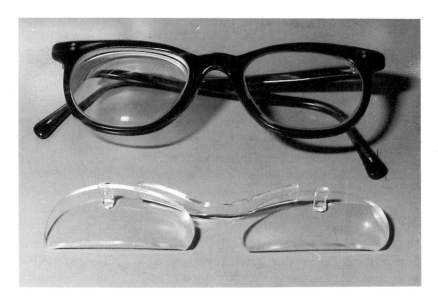

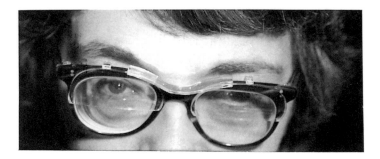

Fig. 14.2 A plastics clip-on constructed with minus spheres for temporary use by a patient with considerable anisometropia. The spectacle frame was glazed with lenses carefully centred for near vision and the added lenses were decentred to minimize vertical prism for distance vision. The device was used to evaluate the possible acceptance of a bifocal correction which might assist binocular vision. Such cases often tend to prefer to alternative the eyes for different modes of vision.

'images' are usually retinal but have been attributed to 'higher' functions producing the discrepancies in percepts. Anisometropia, unilateral aphakia as the outstanding example, as well as the optical magnifications produced by lenses, must be involved.

The patient is likely to experience symptoms which are sometimes difficult to communicate. If binocular vision is seriously attempted there are spatial distortions and difficulties over localisation of objects. It is, for example, a typical cause of complaint if oblique cylinders are altered excessively in power or axis that objects appear skewed and tilted away from the patient. This may be the case even if the astigmatic corrections are 'correct' but the writer was surprised that an investigating committee at which he appeared as 'expert witness' once refused to consider such complaints as valid when a practitioner was accused of incorrect prescribing; it was clear that gross errors had been made, taking older and later optometric prescriptions into account with the patient's reactions. There is a limit to the useful advice 'persevere and you will adapt'.

Retinal size differences over 3 per cent are expected to produce symptoms but there are exceptions. Knapp's law, first enunciated in 1869, appears in most textbooks although the difficulty of determining how much axial length contributes to an individual's ametropia makes the law's application uncertain. Fig. 14.3 gives a slight variation on the usual diagrams which show variations of retinal image size with axial ametropia, whether blurred or corrected in contact with the eye; also how spectacle correction at the anterior focal point influences matters.

In practice aniseikonia is either ignored or, where there is an enthusiast, overemphasized. Hawkswell (1975) provided a simple design for a table-top eikonometer capable of construction by any 'do-it-yourself' amateur as a present-

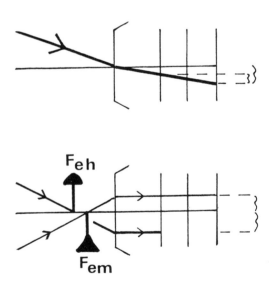

Fig. 14.3 Retinal image sizes with different axial lengths. The reduced eye shown at the top has three possibly lengths; for a given ocular power each produces a different image size, possibly blurred. The lower reduced eye is shown corrected; above there is a hyperopic correction, placed at the anterior focal point, *Feh*, while below a myopic eye is corrected in the same way. The constant image sizes are clearly seen, assuming axial ametropia.

able instrument. Alternatively, the simpler expedient of two point sources viewed direct with one eye and using a Maddox rod in front of the other eye is helpful in 'measuring' relative image sizes. Possibly the tilting plane device is more helpful to a patient who can appreciate your understanding of the problems and your efforts to help with such demonstrations. (See Fig. 14.4.)

A small set of 'size lenses' afocal for distant objects is invaluable. Such can be made up specially as trial lenses, for example giving 1.5, 3 and 6 per cent so that useful combinations can be employed. You can extemporize, combining plus and minus spheres or cyls after the fashion of a Galilean telescope. It is possible to use such lenses with a TIB type chart. There are 'rules of thumb' by which, in a meniscus lens, an increase of − 3.00D in the power of the back surface (BVP being kept constant) can be expected to provide an extra 0.2 per cent

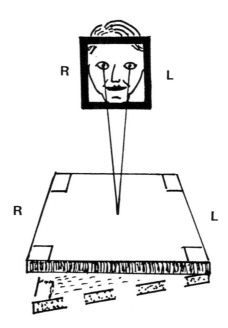

Fig. 14.4 A simple tilting plane for anisoeikonic estimations. With the head fixed the patient looks at a tray or board some 50 cm square, placed horizontally in front of him. A better effect is obtained if a square of fluorescent paper marks each card and a 'black light' near UV source is used in the dark. Tilting of the board is possible, perhaps because it is mounted on four small pillars of clay, so it can be made to appear horizontal to the patient. Suppose the right side must be tilted down to produce an apparently level plane; this would suggest that the left ocular image is relatively large in the vertical meridian, or relatively small horizontally.

magnification per millimetre of thickness. Similarly, each millimetre of extra thickness provides some 0.4 per cent if the back surface power is about $-6.00D$. See also Ryan (1975).

Lens form and vertex distance are the most likely factors to vary in attempts to minimize anisoeikonia; while this approach sometimes involves contact lenses it is often helpful to try the effect of reducing the vertex distance in the more myopic eye, or vice versa and to recognize the effects of 'bending' a lens more or less upon the positions of its principal planes. In the end, some simple eikonometry and practical trials (which should include estimates of stereoscopic vision) have to be the basis of prescribing, hand in glove with dispensing. Adams (1968) gave two very instructive case reports. He showed how one patient was left with a distorted macular image after uniocular macular oedema but was most satisfied with a prescription giving 2 per cent overall magnification with 2½ per cent extra in the vertical meridian. The lens was 6 mm thick, with front surface powers $+11.00D/+5.00D$ and back surface powers $-12.00D/-5.00D$.

14.6   Absorptive lenses

Strictly, 'tinting' of lenses is sometimes replaced or supplemented by coating which alters the reflectance and hence the transmission. Apart from the industrial protective filters (see BS 679, BS 1542, BS 1729 and BS 4808) protective filters for solar radiation are covered in BS 2742. Polarizing filters have advantages in some situations to control reflections which produce glare or reduce visibility, with distinct occupational uses such as swimming pool safety observation. Photophobia is the most likely symptom to raise the question as to whether special absorptive lenses are to be prescribed. There are many causes of the condition, glare being most prevalent, especially in albinism or lightly pigmented persons and in certain situations, perhaps at work in a foundry or during snow or water sports. Ocular disease, such as iritis or conjunctivitis produces photophobia. Mydriasis is a candidate for consideration. The sensory disturbance originates in the iris, the cornea or conjunctival nerves.

Former preoccupation with infra-red and ultraviolet has become modified. This is clear if a comparison of texts is made, such as by Fletcher (1961) and by Miller and Stegmann (1987). The literature and contact lens makers' advertisements have begun to stress the importance of possible damage to the retina from ultraviolet radiation as well as excessive blue light. Aphakics and possibly those with incipient cataract benefit from lenses relatively opaque to ultraviolet and even slight yellow colouration. While neutral density filters are theoretically logical for simple reduction of glare, aesthetic factors intrude and a green filter is probably the best choice for sand and sea. Were the absorption so selective as to lower the visibility of red signals it could be dangerous, but foliage in a barren land tends to assume a refreshing aspect through light green filters. Nevertheless 'brown' lenses have popularity in some quarters and as a compromise between neutral and dark yellow are seldom objectionable. Red and magenta filters, prescribed for Daltonism, as explained in Fletcher and Voke (1985) are valuable for distinct tasks but potentially hazardous for general use and reduction of visibility in tunnels or at night must be pointed out to patients with coloured lenses. The selective absorption of 'sodium light' by Crookes glass filters has been mentioned above but bears repetition here.

Chapter 15
Some Special Patients

While some patients might be called 'difficult' or even 'awkward' one might agree that some optometrists also deserve such a disparaging term, at least at times. So when considering this unusual group of patients who are all out of the ordinary we must be sympathetic, at least. Anyone who appears to present a difficult challenge should prompt us to respond with kindness and efficiency, bringing suitable variations of technique to bear and sometimes asking a colleague to become involved. It is legally possible for you to refuse to accept a patient in the first instance but this must be done with tact and bearing in mind the needs of the patient; presumably someone must accept the challenge. Some situations emerge as difficult after you are committed to caring for an individual. Here you have to do your best, at least for a reasonable time.

It may appear to be unpleasant or unfair to include some types of patient in this section, hence the term 'special'. Special attention is needed by deaf patients as well as by malingerers and unusual features are seldom the patient's 'fault'. I discovered more than once that there are different reasons why someone unhappy with new spectacles deserves careful consideration. More than once an error in dispensing or transposing has happened and once, alas, a colleague actually placed his own similar spectacles near a patient's new ones and the wrong frame was fitted; it was rescued in time.

15.1   Malingering

A patient who wilfully misleads as to the presence or extent of a disability is a 'malingerer'. Duke-Elder (1970) has given a useful review of historic and modern methods of detection. He separated 'simulation' (positive malingering) from 'dissimulation' (negative malingering). The latter applies to someone who memorizes a chart to pretend that form or colour vision is adequate for a desired purpose.

Careful records of all tests are needed. Suspected malingerers' behaviour must be watched carefully, if possible by two people. Behaviour and speech should be encouraged, since either can reveal the situation. It is useful to keep a list so that a variety of tests can be applied rapidly enough to catch the patient off guard.

132

It is rare for total, binocular, blindness to be simulated and such cases are unlikely to appear outside hospital practice. Usually low VA, a field defect or possibly poor dark adaptation is presented. Quietly menacing the face and comparison of pupil reflexes of the two eyes are two of the common approaches to claims of complete blindness. With both eyes open, making rapid horizontal head movements can produce nystagmus in the blind but this result is unlikely if vision is reasonable. Invite the patient to separate the tips of the forefingers, then to touch them rapidly and consider whether any blundering seems to be excessive.

Monocular 'blindness'

Compare objective and subjective prescriptions with various fogging trials, noting their various effects and their relation to pinhole vision.

Overplus the 'good' eye, cover the 'bad' eye and present small letters (which should be seen in focus) to the good eye. As the subject reads on, unobtrusively move the test card away uncovering the 'bad' eye.

Keeping both the eyes open, it is possible to try a variety of ways in which to confuse the patient as to what is being seen by which eye, watching for rapid eye closures. Engage such methods as the FRIEND or FOUR DOT tests, bar reading, a dioploscope with specially reversed symbols and colours; a major amblyoscope can be used, first crossing then uncrossing the tubes and using the switches. If enough tests are used it is likely that you can demonstrate the situation, considering hesitations and changes of opinion, winks and other clues. Plot the blind spot of the good eye while the 'bad' one is open. Fog the good eye by 3DS, record the binocular VA then cover the 'bad' eye and ask whether VA drops.

Assuming that the patient stops at a certain line on the chart, at six metres, it is useful to change to Landolt rings and to alter the viewing distances rapidly; an assistant is helpful here and with the alternation of a direct chart with one seen in a mirror. With care, a tube can be used to restrict the field and clues as to distance. Fahle and Mohn (1989) recommend a preferential looking method with gratings (grey and coloured) which are applied under the pretence of giving a colour vision test. Polarizing filters (opposed) in front of the two eyes can be helpful when charts are projected briefly, through a series of differently orientated polarizing filters.

Using prisms

The prism is an elegant, classical, approach. A fusional movement is to be expected if a suitable prism is placed over a 'bad' eye which has a VA of at least 6/36.

Place a base down prism over a 'blind' eye. Ask if there is diplopia, then make the patient walk rapidly in a complex situation keeping both eyes open.

Prepare a medium power plano prism with a straight edge near the apex, which is placed half over the good pupil, base down, while the 'bad' eye is occluded. Ask if there is diplopia, then continue to discuss the diplopia (and its continuation) as you rapidly remove the occluder and at the same time bring the prism completely over the good pupil.

Hysteria

In such cases complaints are usually binocular and tend to fluctuate. Visual acuity is usually 'poor' but fields of vision can be spiral or reduced, in addition. Prognosis is better in younger patients.

Refer to Slettenberg *et al.* (1989) and to Kramer *et al.* (1979) for modern views.

Are you a capable malingerer?

Please excuse any affront but if you have never tried this spend an hour or so with two colleagues and encourage one to act the part. Remember that most optometrists memorize their charts.

Experience dictates that an umpire is vital.

Of course this is suitable for part of a local Society meeting, if tempers are well under control!

15.2   Communicating with a deaf patient

All patients need careful attention to ensure maximum communication but the deaf present particular needs. It is a great help if a friend or relative comes with the patient and sometimes a local organisation can offer a specialist helper. During and after the examination the reinforcement is useful. The optometrist must make kindly but not condescending efforts to put the patient at ease. It is important to ensure that the patient has several chances to express any worries that arise, for example when, as with some other patients, there is a feeling 'I may have given the wrong answer'. Families greatly appreciate your helpfulness under such circumstances.

The Royal National Institute for the Deaf issues excellent leaflets which give hints, such as *The deaf person in hospital* and *Lip service* but few can become really expert in the special signals used. Do not shout, rather enable the patient to make use of any lip-reading ability by ensuring that your face is visible and in good light. This may include taking account of any 'tunnel' vision introduced by trial lenses or refraction units. Keep still as you speak, using clear but not exaggerated lip movements and speak fairly slowly. Smile in all the right places. Be ready to note lack of understanding, when you must repeat yourself using different words. Use definite but fairly short sentences. Employ simple hand signals, such as 'thumbs up', but with discretion. Do ensure that your lips are visible, not covered by a hand or instrument as you speak.

Some optometrists prepare cards with clear 'key questions' or instructions; for example 'which lens is better, FIRST or SECOND?'. Writing on a pad can help, even one of the techniques of 'writing' on the patient's hand with your finger. This method is particularly used for the deaf-blind, which can include those with partial sight and the Royal National Institute for the Blind supplies a small card with ideas on using it. For example, you form the letter T with two strokes or N with a zig-zag stroke. Using your own trained assistant is a great help. Allow extra time. The appreciation and success resulting from such efforts are very rewarding, as is your increased confidence on your retinoscopic prowess and such experiences certainly relieve any tedium in practice.

15.3 Domiciliary visits

Housebound patients, or those unable to visit you if your rooms are upstairs, need professional attention in their own homes. Arrange for a relative or friend to be present or for a lady colleague to accompany a male optometrist. Well in advance, clarify the fullest details of the patient's situation, history and records, plus the way in which fees are to be met.

A few mentally handicapped adults are anxious or frightened if they are seen in your practice, mistaking the place for a dental surgery with its attendant memories! A home visit can then be the only way you can help.

Prepare a portable kit, including a small set of trial lenses, optotypes and a portable tonometer (see Fig. 15.1). Remember spare batteries for your instruments and include a torch which can be useful for negotiating dark stairs or for heterophorias. Take a compact desk lamp with a 100-watt bulb, some partial sight aids and some suitable frames. You may have to attempt running repairs, needing screwdrivers, pins, pliers, screws, lens packing, instant glues and adhesive tape. Be prepared to offer instant acceptable occlusion for diplopia, to demonstrate basic filters or to show the benefit of extra illumination. A collapsible centimetre rule serves for siting charts and for accommodation measurements.

It is difficult to resist the temptation to rehearse certain vivid memories of domiciliary visits, some requiring rubber boots to reach farms where the test chart had to be held outside an open door to provide enough illumination. Further temptation is resisted. Be prepared to have a door key thrown from above by a bedridden pensioner. Your visit may be such an event that you have to devote time to chatting. Be discerning over offered refreshments.

15.4 Complaints

Sometimes the valid cause of a patient's complaints about new spectacles is an inaccurate prescription. For example, among almost two thousand patients Cockburn (1987) found almost 6 per cent who were given a new prescription

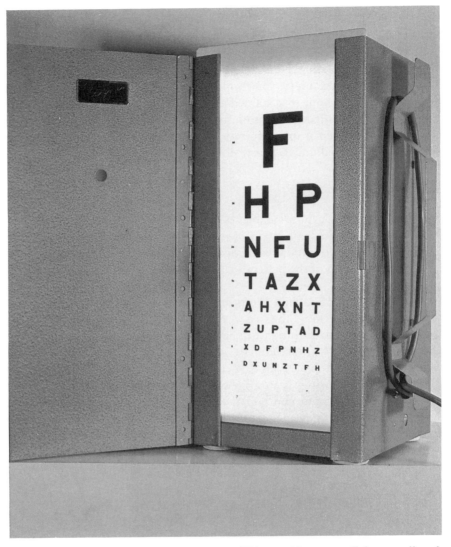

Fig. 15.1 Portable internally illuminated chart. This provides a spot light as well as letter charts. For the completely equipped domiciliary visitor. (Courtesy of Rayner Optical Co.)

voicing difficulties within two months. His paper is valuable for new optometrists. Of the 53 patients who complained, 15 were discovered to have been given spectacles which could be improved. Some had excessive plus sphere, some had been given too little and ten of the situations could be blamed on 'unsatisfactory communication' with patients. There were seven anisoeikonias which distorted images. For seven patients the cause of the difficulty remained a mystery.

Cockburn pointed out that some people believe that incorrect lenses can damage their sight. Some do not return to complain. It is a delicate decision whether encouraging patients to return if they have any difficulty tends to inspire confidence or suggests that difficulty is likely. Almost half of those who complained, in Cockburn's series, had earlier been noted to be 'unreliable' in their responses. (See Chapter 19, cases 15 and 16.)

Chapter 16
Accessories used in Ocular Refraction

During student days collections of instruments are started, ranging from ophthalmoscopes to small engraved paddles used for cover testing or near points of convergence. Emerging into practice, often having to work with unfamiliar equipment, or moving around between practices the new optometrist tends to add several small but valuable accessories. This short account emphasizes some personal preferences.

Standard items are part of most trial cases and refraction units, in addition to lenses. The selection of occluders, pinholes and slits does make one wonder, at times, whether the designers had tried to use any of these. Maddox multiple grooves are commonplace but at times the single 'rod' cylinder appears, making observation just a little more difficult for most patients. One seldom sees a cobalt blue plano filter nowadays, although it was the origin of bichromatic tests but few would seek one. The urge to start a personal collection of small aids to refraction usually starts with pinholes; for some reason very small apertures are often supplied making it necessary to attack them with a penknife before they are useful.

Possession of several empty trial lens rims and a supply of white, grey or black thin styrene sheet is a good start. The sheet is found in model shops and discs are easily scored with a pair of dividers, allowing easy extrusion of the shape by finger pressure. Handles are easily stuck on with the appropriate cement so a range of devices from multiple pinholes to 'typoscope' aids for reading can be constructed.

16.1 Pinholes

It is easy to glaze standard rims, or discs can be made to fit trial cells, unrimmed. Ideally central apertures of 1.5 mm, 2 mm, 2.5 mm and even 3 mm can be drilled, making a valuable set. The most useful is often 2 mm diameter. Spares are essential!

Often a large disc is convenient for a patient to hold, containing a single pinhole or a simple pattern of holes which allows rapid location of one. Such discs should have handles attached so that patients can manipulate the device. Clip-on or stick-on pinhole attachments are very useful for partial sight cases. Fig. 16.1 illustrates an Italian product which can be cut to size and stuck on. The author's

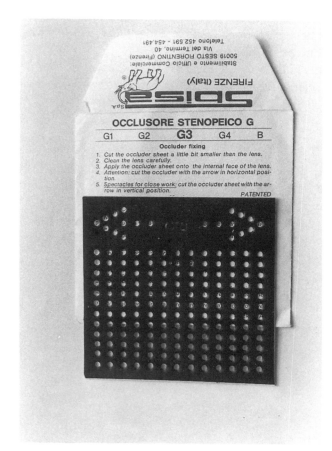

Fig. 16.1 Stenopaeic pinhole sheets. These are supplied with a self adhesive backing and are cut to fit the whole or part of a spectacle lens. The holes shown are 3 mm in diameter and are spaced differently along two axes. For reading use, the orientation is so that the larger spaces are disposed vertically.

father frequently made opaque discs with multiple holes for patients, mounted as zinc sheet alternatives to lenses or as 'over spectacles' and many were of great benefit.

Stenopaeic slits in different widths are handy for some difficult situations and may be made in sets comprising 1.5 mm, 2 mm and 3 mm.

16.2 Occluders

Translucent or at least white material is sometimes preferred since patients may feel less constricted than with truly opaque occlusion during refraction. Some materials avoid a consensual pupil dilation. Pirate patches in fabric are less hygienic than plastics domes often used in field plotting and some are held by a spring. A tissue beneath adds to comfort and a sense of greater hygienic care but pressure on the globe should be avoided.

When patients hold the occluder ensure that there is neither peeping nor such massive thrust against the cornea that the occluded eye takes a while to recover.

16.3   Prisms

Remarkably, the Risley prism is seldom used, except when fitted to refraction units. Often the bulk and the small aperture make the gadget difficult to use but it is worth having.

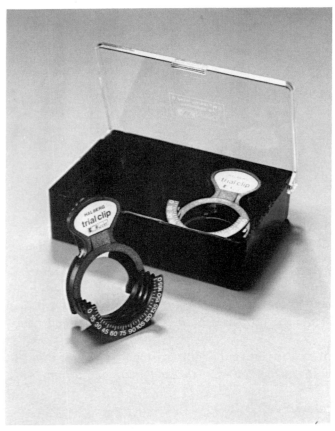

Fig. 16.2   Halberg trial clips. Invaluable for holding a variety of temporary lenses/discs, they must be placed and retained on a spectacle lens with care. (Courtesy of Keeler Ltd.)

A separate 3 prism dioptre (pd) plano prism is valuable; since trial lenses have small handles it should be mounted like a crossed cylinder but with the base–apex line at 45 degrees to the handle, allowing it to be twirled. Holding this base in, for example, combined with a Maddox rod, one can move the handle nearer to the vertical to introduce variable prism effects in vertical and horizontal meridians allowing neat rapid estimates of heterophorias. With the handle at 180 the vertical and horizontal components are about 1.5 pd.

In practice a large round eye metal clip-on frame is an excellent way to experiment with prism corrections. Glaze with 3 pd meniscus afocal lenses and mark the bases inconspicuously. The rims can be unscrewed slightly to allow the prism effects to be altered. Using 3 pd R and L it is possible to range from 6 pd base in to 6 base out; also starting with one base in along 180 and the other out along 180, a series of vertical alternative prism powers can be produced.

The use of a trial clip (Fig. 16.2) monocularly or binocularly is another way to provide temporary prism power, provided the stability of the clips on spectacle frames is ensured.

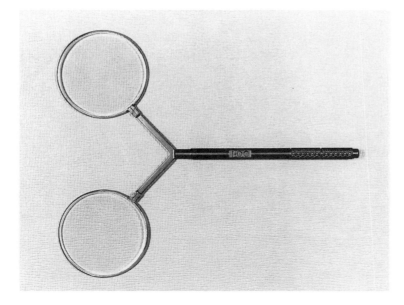

Fig. 16.3 Binocular addition. In this case both lenses are + 1.00DS. The device can be adapted to hold plus and minus lenses on each side. (Courtesy of Rayner Optical Co.)

16.4   Binocular additions

Spherical binocular additions, mounted in the lorgnette type of frame shown in Figs. 16.3 and 16.4 are useful in refraction and when demonstrating the depth of field with different additions. Centres are usually 62 mm apart, the lenses being meniscus. The most useful powers are R and L + 0.50D, + 1.00DS, + 1.50DS, + 2.00DS, − 0.50DS and − 0.75DS. The minus powers are excellent for demonstrating 'night' myopia, so an extra pair of − 0.75DS lenses with AR coating might be added to the set, as a clip-on, for temporary trial by patients under 'working conditions'. The plus binocular additions serve also to show the advantages of lorgnettes for shopping or lecturing in suitable cases.

16.5   Bifocal demonstration sets

At least one manufacturer of multifocal lenses issues a comprehensive set of demonstration lenses, with a special skeleton frame. Pairs of ordinary size trial

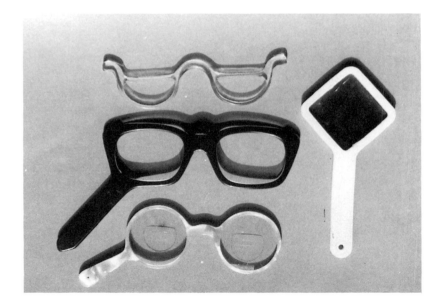

Fig. 16.4   A range of accessories. At the top a 'slip-in' intermediate or reading addition frame, placed temporarily behind a distance spectacle frame. Below this is a typical binocular addition mount in lorgnette form. Underneath a pair of 'D' segment straight top bifocals is seen, mounted in a lorgnette. At the right is a single filter holder in which thin filters can be protected between cover glasses, used for daylight conversion from tungsten and a variety of alternatives.

rims should also be considered, glazed with some 'inset' as R and L lenses, using powers such as + 0.75DS, + 1.25DS, + 1.75DS, + 2.25DS and + 2.75DS, with a pair of + 4.50DS for special purposes. Ideally, medium-size straight top segments should be used. A smaller set of a typical progressive lens form will be a great help. All these lenses, with afocal distance portions, are very convincing to patients who are uncertain as to the advantages of multifocals. A lorgnette mount for a pair of bifocals of this type is illustrated in Fig. 16.4.

16.6   Special attachments

As already shown in Fig. 14.2 there is much scope for ingenuity and extemporization for certain needs. One patient had unusual difficulties when walking with bifocals but since she addressed meetings frequently and required rapid alternation between her distance hyperopic correction and an intermediate presbyopic addition, considered a lorgnette; this she felt to appear as an affectation and a compromise, seen at the top of Fig. 16.4, was completely successful. A half-eye frame was made with lugs which supported the addition on the sides of the

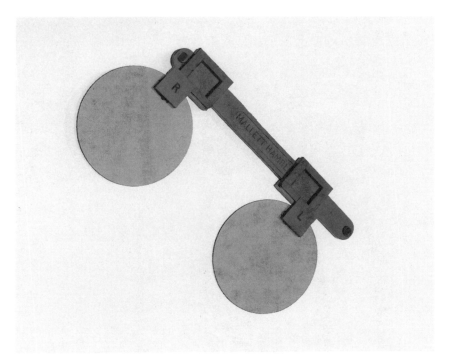

Fig. 16.5 'Crossed' polarizing filters, suspended in front of the trial lenses. Note the variable separation. Ensure that the planes of polarization match the orientations of test chart filters. (Courtesy of Keeler Ltd.)

spectacle, having slipped the 'half-eye' behind the distance spectacles. This permitted removal and satisfactory mobility after the address.

Monocles, rather like half-eye frames, tend to add a theatrical air but have immense practical uses in the right cases. While such devices are intimately concerned with the dispensing of a prescription there is no reason why a prescriber who does not do the dispensing should not enter into full discussion of possibilities, when suitable adjustments to powers may be indicated.

A plastics clip-on binocular addition for librarians and storekeepers is available (C.O.I.L.) in which half-eye lenses are held above the centre of the spectacle lenses. Painters and some aircrew personnel can use this, particularly when there is doubt as to the optimum power and position of the addition for their special needs and some practical trial will help.

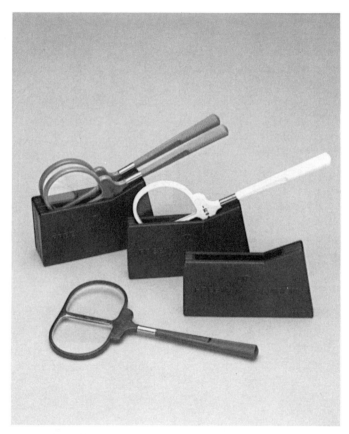

Fig. 16.6 Plus and minus 'flip' holders in different powers, colour coded. (Courtesy of Keeler Ltd.)

16.7   Miscellaneous items

The polarizing attachments shown in Fig. 16.5 are found in slightly different forms, sometimes with vertically and horizontally orientated planes of polarization, alternatively with 45 and 135 orientations in the two lenses. A large single polarizing filter mounted in combination with a blue (such as Lee Filters 132 Medium Blue, Y value approximately 8 per cent) is fine to permit patients to observe Haidinger's brushes for macular assessment.

Bagolini striated lenses are produced with careful application of strokes of abrasive paper to plastics or glass discs or by grease wiped across a surface. Lee Filters 228 Brushed Silk filter gives a strong linear image of a spot light. All such

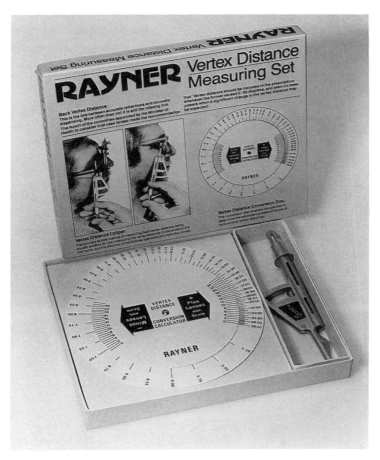

Fig. 16.7   Vertex distance device, with calculator disc for effective powers. (Courtesy of Rayner Optical Co.)

items should be sandwiched between covers of glass or plastics. Thin plastics filters can be mounted instead of transparency prints in 35 mm slide mounts or the thin glass can be adapted for covers.

Red and blue-green complementary filters are essential for dissociation and use with malingerers, etc. Lee Filters 119 Dark Blue, or 120 Deep Blue, are splendid for Maxwell's spot observations and their range of Neutral Density Filters is suitable for many consulting room uses; when using polarized light neutrals made of gelatine may be required.

Lee Filters supply large sheets of blue filters which can be adapted for converting tungsten light to approximate daylight, such as 201 Full CT Blue and 202 ½ CT Blue.

Sets of 'flip' holders with suitable alternative lenses such as ±0.25DS are invaluable aids, see Fig. 16.6. Every practice needs accurate means of measuring vertex distances after refractions and after dispensing, such as the device shown in Fig. 16.7. Last, but hardly least and remarkably helpful as part of the domiciliary outfit, there is a need for a test chart which permits a standard measure of vision and visual acuity.

Part 3
Cases
D C STILL

Chapter 17
Advice to Younger Colleagues

This third part, on refraction and subjective examination, is intended to assist newcomers to optometry to obtain a clearer idea of the actual tasks facing them and to help to develop confidence in their prescribing. The main intention is to provide a practical 'hands-on' approach to the work. It is not proposed to go into elaborate details of the theory behind the techniques described, though some explanations will be given.

The methods used for ascertaining the refractive error in everyday practice, and the problems likely to arise in straightforward refraction, will be discussed in some detail, but considerable space will also be devoted to a wide selection of cases – varying from the commonplace to the rare – which draw attention to special difficulties which may need to be considered in regard to preliminary assessment, examination or prescribing. All the examples given are real, and have been taken from the writer's own extensive record files which extend over a period of about 40 years.

No pretence of superiority or infallibility is made when advocating what is considered to be the best course to take in any given example. The reader may well reason out different or better solutions for some of the prescribing problems described. There is often more than one possible answer, and it must be recognized that even the best solution often involves a compromise.

Instances of faulty prescribing and dispensing have also been included. These also are all real! (A few of them have been the subject of complaints made by patients which resulted in referral to an Ophthalmic Investigation Committee for assessment and re-examination where members considered it to be justified). In some instances the errors were due to an individual's lack of experience, but in others they probably arose because insufficient time and thought had been given to the problems involved. It is hoped that the inclusion of such examples will help the practitioner to avoid some of the mistakes that can all too easily occur.

The newly qualified should not feel daunted by the number of different things to be considered when undertaking the prescribing of spectacles. When actually faced with a problem case, a practical and logical plan of action is essential; one has to learn how to make an objective assessment of the whole situation, and apply tests to eliminate the various possible causative factors until those responsible have been isolated. A few of the cases will seem tedious and obvious to experienced practitioners, but these have been included for the benefit of the newly qualified individual who is only just beginning to get involved in the problems of everyday practice.

17.1   The work environment

Young practitioners who have just left university have been used to using high quality equipment, usually up-to-date and regularly serviced, and have been encouraged to spend adequate time developing the skills they need, but the realities of professional practice can be a disturbing experience. They may be fortunate enough to enter a prestigious practice with magnificent equipment, helpful and considerate colleagues, in which they are under no pressure to streamline their techniques, but it is more likely that they will have to settle for something less exciting.

If on the other hand, they encounter gross inefficiency, aggressive and critical colleagues or staff, and find they have to use old or unfamiliar equipment, they should endeavour to remain calm and wait until they have begun to comprehend the organization and routine (what industrial psychologists call 'maze awareness'), when they will very likely find the circumstances more tolerable than at first imagined. They should also bear in mind that they may have some minor faults that an employer finds irritating but thinks it wiser to overlook at this early stage. (For example 'He doesn't switch the lights/instruments off'. 'She never cleans her fingerprints off the trial lenses', or 'He never puts things away when he's finished with them', etc.)

Most practices are far better equipped today than they were some years ago, but the variations and layout can differ so widely that great versatility is required when moving from one practice to another. The layout may have been constrained by economic and structural factors – I recall a test-room in an expensive London area, for instance, where a direct chart was used, but with *two* mirrors, so that the required six-metre length could be obtained in a confined space. Or the whole set-up may have been devised for a left-handed individual, which can be most disconcerting initially. A minority of practices, it must be admitted, are just so badly arranged that it seems incredible that no effort has been made to make at least a few simple alterations that would have greatly improved working conditions.

A few actual examples may be of interest here; some of them I have seen for myself, others have been described to me by younger members of the profession, together with the methods they adopted to cope with the problems, which give some indication of the degree of adaptability required.

1   'The spotlight is so low that the patient's head usually comes in front of it, and he can't see it in the mirror'. It was not possible to move the patient's chair, so

pending a proper solution of this difficulty dynamic retinoscopy was performed, the patient being directed to look at a distance test letter during the final stages. The ophthalmoscope was used as a spotlight for Maddox rod tests.

2 'My duochrome test is useless. The red filter has a ridiculously low transmission compared with the green'. This practitioner developed a technique of estimating the sphere as accurately as possible by retinoscopy, and using this as the basis for using the cross-cylinder. For binocular balancing he used a polaroid test or alternate monocular occlusion.

3 'My test chart (which includes an astigmatic fan) is set on the patient's left, with its centre at about the level of his head. The trial case and hand instruments are all on his right. It might be tolerable if I had a remote control mechanism for the switches, but I have to keep getting up and leaning across the patient to reach them'. The only short cuts possible here were to leave several panels illuminated, and to use the cross-cylinder in preference to the fan chart.

Numerous other criticisms of the layout and apparatus provided could be cited. Often they were valid, but in some instances they were simply due to lack of familiarity with a particular instrument or technique. That is why it is wiser to suspend judgement until one has settled in. The proprietor of the practice may have been too worried or too busy to sit back and think how best to reorganize his methods of working, and might be glad to have some helpful suggestions. There is no doubt at all that one can do a better and more productive job if the working environment is comfortable and the equipment and controls easily accessible.

17.2 Professional freedom

More important than the work environment is the need for genuine professional freedom. There is no point in having an impressive array of equipment, for instance, unless sufficient time is allowed to make good use of it. One has to be realistic, of course, because economic and practical factors have to be taken into account. But for the enthusiastic optometrist, job satisfaction must have a high priority, and one of the cardinal principles to be borne in mind is that *good work takes time*. I regard this dictum as so important that, even if it is the only message the reader can recall after reading this book, I shall not feel that my efforts have been entirely wasted.

17.3 Entering a new practice

It will be a great advantage to the optometrist embarking on his career if he enjoys dealing with people and is able to get on with them. It should not need to be said, but unfortunately it often does, that when an individual first arrives at a new, or different, place of work he should be sure to greet the existing staff pleasantly, and to try to remember their names. He may be asked if he would rather be called, say,

Fred, or Mr Smith, and the decision calls for just a little care. (Readers must appreciate that wherever they see 'he' the writer obviously intends 'he or she'; he is well aware of the high percentage of female optometrists!) It is generally more pleasant to be on first-name terms, but it can add to your difficulties if you find yourself left in charge of staff who are much older than you are and who may be uncooperative.

A common grievance among new entrants to a practice is that it has not been made clear to them precisely what their duties are. Generally speaking, in a small but busy practice, one simply looks round to see what needs to be done and gets on with it if time allows, whether it happens to be checking, adjustments, minor repairs, or whatever. With larger organizations, particularly those with multiple outlets, functions and responsibilities are more clearly defined. Some optometrists consider that their responsibilities should be limited only to examination and refraction ('the job I was trained to do'). But a wider acquaintance with the varied aspects of running a practice is an excellent experience – certainly a tremendous advantage if you want to run your own some day.

17.4   Familiarize yourself with the equipment

It is highly important to familiarize yourself with the equipment and layout of the test room you are going to use before commencing any examinations. Try out the switches, check through the instruments to see that they are set up and working properly, and make sure you know how to adjust the patient's chair. If there is a refractor head and it is not the type you are used to, spend a few minutes learning how to manipulate it with reasonable confidence. If you are to use a trial case, check out the steps available in spheres and cylinders, and the range of accessories. Be sure you can find the occluder, and don't mix it up with the pinhole disc, or you will find your first case more challenging than you had imagined. If these preliminaries are ignored, the first few patients you see will notice your clumsiness and hesitation and are likely to lose confidence in your ability. I recall having to take over from a colleague on one occasion at extremely short notice, in a practice I had not visited before. Within moments of my arrival the first patient was shown in, for which I was unprepared. I had not at this stage been given a record card, and he had already been waiting for some time, so I commenced taking case history details and performed some preliminary tests. I then made the unfortunate mistake of asking him 'Have you been here before', to which he replied 'Yes, many times. Have you?'

17.5   General routines

Find out who is expected to fill out preliminary details on the record cards, and whether you are expected to show the patient into the test room or one of the staff, and what the facilities are for dispensing when necessary. Never be afraid to ask. The practices which provide the least advice and training are often those in which resentment or jealousy are most likely to arise through misunderstandings.

Many practices now employ a dispenser, but if you are required to attend to this yourself you will need a *considerable* amount of time to scrutinise the various manufacturers' lists, to get used to the enormous range of lenses, tints, and frames available, and to acquaint yourself with the methods of pricing. Dispensing is much more complicated than is often supposed – don't ever disparage it – the technical expertise required for good work demands respect and if it is not carried out intelligently the results of the most careful refraction can be sabotaged. For this reason, although dispensing is outside the scope of this volume, examples will be given in instances where it can affect the work of the optometrist, especially in regard to 'grief cases'. Remember that a refraction performed is not finished when the prescription is issued. It has then to be translated into the end product of a frame and lenses, and fitted to the patient.

If this end product proves unsatisfactory, complaints may initially be addressed to the dispenser. If difficulty persists, they are then transferred to a prescriber (not necessarily the original prescriber), who must be prepared to unravel the cause of the trouble, which may arise from the prescription, the lens form or weight, the fitting, or even the psychology of the wearer, among other things. This can be a challenging and time-consuming exercise, requiring much patience, especially if the prescription is recent, and originated with another optometrist.

Dealing with complaints and difficulties has always formed a relatively small but very significant part of the optometrist's duties, and it is recently beginning to assume greater importance. For many years all patients in the UK were entitled to a free eye examination, and if they were dissatisfied with the spectacles supplied the prescriber would often apply to have the lenses altered and replaced at no charge under the 'non-tolerance' rules of the National Health Service. Or the patient could arrange to consult another practitioner for a further opinion without charge after a relatively short waiting period, and obtain new lenses if a change was made in the prescription.

These facilities have now largely been rescinded, and optometrists are discovering that clients who complain are becoming tougher and more persistent now that they have to pay. I have heard colleagues complain, in effect, that people seem to be getting nastier nowadays, but their surprise simply reflects the fact that we have as a profession enjoyed an easy ride because of the relatively benevolent NHS regulations referred to; they are only experiencing the normal reactions of members of the public when they feel, rightly or wrongly, that they have not been given a fair deal.

Chapter 18
First Steps prior to Examination

18.1   Sit the patient comfortably

Having acquainted yourself with the general layout and organization of the practice, you should now be ready to see your first patient for consultation.

Greet patients when they enter the consulting room, show them where to put down any items they are carrying, so that you do not inadvertently tread on them when the lights are turned out, and make sure that they are sitting comfortably in the chair. If it is an adjustable or hydraulic chair it must be set to the correct height and facing squarely towards the test chart or mirror. Remember the head rest, which should be set at the appropriate angle at the junction of the head and neck.

(Some head rests are most unsatisfactory, as they cannot be raised sufficiently to suit the patient of average height, and lack any form of forward adjustment. If this applies to the one you have been given to use, there is no point in spending too much time trying to get it right.)

The foot rest, if fitted and of the fixed type, can be a nuisance to old, crippled, or unsteady persons, who may have difficulty in stepping up. On the other hand, if the chair you are using is of a design which permits it to be swung temporarily out of the way, remember to turn it back after the patient is settled in, or he will be left with his legs dangling uncomfortably in mid-air.

18.2   Preliminary assessment

The initial examination and case history taking may provide clues to possible changes in refraction, and to the expected corrected acuity. Obvious examples are the schoolchild who has recently had difficulty in seeing the blackboard – probably low myopia; or the 40-year-old who now finds it necessary to hold work further out – early presbyopia. Ophthalmoscopy will have shown if defects such as cataract, corneal scarring, or macular changes are present, while the powers racked into the sighthole can also give a rough guide to the type of refractive error. The 'expected acuity' is important because, if vision cannot be improved to somewhere near the level anticipated, it will be advisable to check back to ensure that nothing has been missed.

154

Patients should be 'talked to', particularly at the first meeting, to put them at their ease and to assess their visual needs or difficulties. A little time spent at this stage can produce valuable information, and may indicate the best way to proceed. Look at them when you first greet them as they enter the room, and make them feel welcome. The modern practitioner must learn to be observant, and will soon come to realize that the very first impressions can be informative; signs such as strabismus or ptosis may be observed, for instance.

In fact, an intelligent appraisal will occasionally reveal significant signs even before the patient has spoken to you, as the following examples illustrate.

1   The pupils are seen to be greyish, and not black, even on cursory inspection. Or dense corneal scarring may be visible. This is a good indication that the task ahead is certainly going to be difficult, and quite likely impossible. If the patient complains that his old glasses have never been any good the optometrist will know that it is highly unlikely that he will be able to supply anything better, and will colour his responses accordingly.

2   As this patient entered the room I was struck by his exceptionally tall, gangling appearance. As he sat down he placed his long, large hands on the arms of the refraction chair. This was the first hint that he might possibly be affected with Marfan's syndrome. Looking at his eyes, irido-donesis could be discerned before any examination was commenced, indicating that this was indeed the case, so that ectopia lentis, which usually accompanies this condition would be present, together with all the attendant problems of prescribing, of course.

3   An elderly patient, walking through the consulting room doorway, was observed to put out his hand to feel for the door frame on one side. The immediate reaction should be 'I wonder if perhaps he's got a field defect on that side'. And, it transpired, so he had; he had a severe limitation which was found to be due to previously undiagnosed glaucoma.

4   The spectacles worn are seen to be badly fitting or bent, suggesting a very simple reason for ocular discomfort if no change is found in the refraction.

18.3   Who is watching whom?

Remember that just as you are assimilating your first impressions of the patient, he is likewise forming his first impressions about you. Never adopt an impersonal or offhand manner, which is a sure way of encouraging antagonism and resentment. It need hardly be said that the professional man or woman should look reasonably neat and clean; one is not required to be a model of sartorial elegance, but a scruffy appearance is more likely to inspire criticism than confidence. The best results are obtained from consultations where the patient is relaxed, is treated politely, and feels he or she is being encouraged to co-operate. Incidentally all patients, except friends or children, must in general be addressed as Mr or Mrs X and never treated patronizingly. Sometimes a younger relative brings in an aged patient whose faculties are beginning to fail. So far as is possible your questions should be addressed to the patients themselves; don't talk over their heads to the relatives unless you are unable to get satisfactory replies.

Similarly, if you are dealing with a complaint, bear in mind that what may seem absurdly trivial or frivolous to you may genuinely worry some people. One of the commonest objections comes from presbyopic patients, who say that their distance vision is blurred when they are wearing their reading glasses. The fact that this is patently obvious to the prescriber does not give him the right to treat it dismissively; he could in any case have anticipated the question and mentioned it at the time of the examination. These patients will often insist that they could always see at distance with their old reading glasses, which calls for a brief explanation of the inevitable onset of presbyopia with advancing age.

Another complaint that may at first baffle the inexperienced is that of 'I get a blur wherever I look', or 'There's a flaw in my lenses'.

Inspection reveals that they are in perfect condition, and it may be some time before it is realized that the trouble is 'only' due to reflections from the lens surfaces. Fortunately this is heard less frequently nowadays, with the greater use of anti-reflection coatings. Nevertheless, a few patients seem to be unduly disturbed by these reflections, and if they are persistent, the front should be angled back slightly, which may make them less obtrusive.

18.4   What was the previous prescription?

If spectacles are already worn, ask to see the latest pairs if they are available. It is advisable – almost mandatory – to ascertain the old prescription, though one must not be unduly influenced by it, or allow oneself to be too impressed by the status of the previous prescriber. In particular, *it should never be assumed that the old cylinders and axes are probably about right*, and that one could chance putting them into the trial frame and simply modify the sphere. We all come across evidence of such short cuts on occasions, and the results are often disastrous. When the old glasses are focimetered, either by yourself or by an assistant, ensure that the centration, together with the bifocal segment inset if applicable, is included with the prescription, as it may have constituted a source of trouble. Also, if you insist that the centration is put down, it may warn you that circumspection will be needed if it differs appreciably from that indicated by the interpupillary distance, and it is also much less likely that any prism incorporated will be overlooked.

This is very important. There are no hard and fast rules for the prescribing of prisms, and the methods used vary with the individual practitioner, but there is no doubt that (provided they have been intelligently assessed) some patients derive enormous benefit from them. Trouble can arise either because (a) they had been worn before and you had not noticed, or had not thought them to be necessary, or (b) although you have given proper consideration to the binocular status and decided to give them, the patient had not worn them before and cannot tolerate their inclusion. Actual instances are cited below which illustrate these points very well.

An investigation

This case came under the jurisdiction of an Ophthalmic Investigation Committee. The patient was new to the optometrist who examined him, who noted early lens changes which produced scissor-like reflexes in retinoscopy which were difficult to interpret; he attempted to make an assessment with an auto-refractor, but results were again not satisfactory. He prescribed:

> R $-0.50/-0.75 \times 110$
> L $-2.25/-2.75 \times 105$
> Add $+2.75$ reading

These were made up as varifocal spectacles, but the patient was unable to get on with them, and returned several times, complaining of overlapping images with his left eye and double vision. He then visited another practitioner, who ordered a very similar prescription but incorporated 1^{Δ} base down in the right eye, and 1^{Δ} base up in the left. When this was dispensed it was quite satisfactory, but the irate patient wished to recuperate the cost of the first prescription and registered an official complaint.

At the hearing it was easy to verify that appreciable lens changes were present, and also that monocular diplopia was present with his left eye, which had tended to confuse the problem. The refractive correction was confirmed, but in spite of the lens changes his visual acuity did not fall far short of 6/6. There was about $2\frac{1}{2}^{\Delta}$ of R. hyperphoria present (which of course justified the prisms), and it was discovered that similar prisms had been included in the prescription he had been wearing prior to that which had given rise to the dispute.

The practitioner concerned admitted that he had not measured the muscle balance; possibly he would have thought to do this on the latest appointment he had arranged for a further recheck, but by this time the patient had decided he had had enough; he cancelled the appointment and went elsewhere for a complete reassessment.

Hyperphoria

This patient, a man of 40, had a much higher degree of hyperphoria, varying around 9^{Δ}. His prescription was:

> R $+6.00/-2.00 \times 120$ 6/9 $+2\frac{1}{2}^{\Delta}$ base down
> L $+6.00/-2.25 \times 50$ 6/9 $+2\frac{1}{2}^{\Delta}$ base up

He had no difficulty wearing this, but was persuaded, about a year later, to consult another practitioner, when new spectacles were prescribed. As soon as he collected them, he complained that he was getting double vision (for the very obvious reason that the prisms had been omitted) but he was 'reassured' that he would get used to them. He was most annoyed, and would not on any account return to this individual (who probably regarded the case as successful as he did not get further complaints), but visited the original prescriber, who found the prescription would have been quite satisfactory if the prisms had been retained.

Dissatisfaction

In this case the patient, a man of about 50 with approximately 1.25DS of hypermetropia, did not have prisms incorporated in his existing lenses, but he consulted a different optometrist, who said he found 4^Δ R hyperphoria and 4^Δ esophoria at distance. Though there was little change in the basic prescription, he felt justified in correcting this, as there was a complaint of ocular discomfort and from other tests he performed he thought prisms would be beneficial.

Unfortunately, the patient took his prescription elsewhere to have it dispensed, but found the spectacles were uncomfortable and made his eyes ache. He did not go back to the original prescriber, who would probably have modified the prescription to satisfy him, but sought another opinion. He was then prescribed new spectacles, without the prisms, which he found perfectly comfortable.

This case also went to an Ophthalmic Investigation Committee hearing, at which two independent optometrists were invited to examine the patient. The degrees of heterophoria found were exactly as had been stated, though the patient did not really seem to notice whether prisms were put in or not, when he was viewing the distance chart binocularly. It was observed that he had a scar under his left eye, which he dismissed as just an old injury he had suffered some 20 years before. This had probably damaged the L inferior oblique, which subsequent tests revealed was the muscle at fault.

Further tests showed that he had about 6^Δ of excyclophoria, confirming the suspicion that there was a tendency to central suppression with the left eye. If this had not been present he would have been likely to experience asthenopia whatever lenses were prescribed.

Misalignment

It should be evident that hyperphoria can be produced artificially in anisometropia, if the optical centres of the lenses have not been properly adjusted to the level of the pupils. But even if the lens powers are practically the same, similar difficulties can arise.

A lady patient, who had been seen regularly, had the following prescription:

R + 5.75/ − 1.00   80 2$^\Delta$ base up
L + 5.50/ − 1.00   85
2$^\Delta$ L Hyperphoria Ortho. H distance

The right eye was set a full 3 mm higher than the left, thus inducing a base-down right-eye effect from the effective difference in centration of the trial lenses. For many years this had been allowed for in dispensing her spectacles, and when she became presbyopic the required effect was obtained by appropriate setting of her bifocals. Not long after this examination she decided to attend another optometrist for advice, who arrived at the correct basic correction, but failed to notice the difference in eye level. (Yes, if only he had looked at the old lenses, it would have alerted him to this factor.)

Not surprisingly, the spectacles were unsatisfactory, and she returned to her original prescriber for advice. It was noticed that she was wearing the frame tilted down to the left, and she said she had discovered they seemed more comfortable like this. The reason should be evident to the reader, and she might well have tolerated this expedient for longer, but they had been dispensed as flat-top bifocals with the same segment height on each lens.

18.5   Prescribing prisms

The above examples should not give the refractionist any cause for anxiety regarding the prescribing of prisms; they should simply serve as a warning that care and thought has to be given to each individual case, in addition to the tests you have applied which have convinced you of their need.

Ensure that the trial frame is level and properly centred, and check to see if binocular vision is present. Always let the patient wear the prisms you are proposing to prescribe for at least a few moments before you write down your prescription on the record card. Generally speaking, if the prism is necessary, the patient will often report immediate improvement or relief or at the very least he will not voice any objection. If he or she frowns, or reacts in some disapproving way, check first that you have set the base in the correct direction. Bear in mind what he/she has been wearing before, and take another look at the old prescription if the results do not seem to support your conclusions.

With regard to cyclophoria, this does deserve a brief mention. Many optometrists virtually never look for this, considering it too rare to bother about and in any case not treatable. However, if an oblique muscle paresis is suspected – as, for example, in the section 'Dissatisfaction' above – checks should be made for possible associated cyclophoria. With torsional errors of this degree the patient may complain persistently of eyestrain and discomfort if normal binocular vision is present. It is therefore preferable to detect it at the time of the examination, *before* any complaint is made. When a problem can be explained in advance the patient will be more willing to accept it.

18.6   Bifocal tolerance

It has already been mentioned that patients often return with seemingly trivial complaints. Bifocals are a particular source of difficulty; many individuals are not prepared to make any effort to adapt to them, and will return with them even if they have been accurately fitted but set fractionally higher or lower than they have been accustomed to. A frequent complaint arises when the reading addition has been increased, for instance, from + 1.25DS to + 1.75DS – enough to blur the ground in front of them slightly more, and making them feel unsteady. Arguments over this point can become quite acrimonious ('My old pair never blurred me up like this', they say), and the optometrist may need all the tact and patience he can muster to settle what he may regard as merely one of the inevitable minor disadvantages of advancing presbyopia.

On the other hand, it is equally extraordinary to discover the extent to which some other patients can learn to adapt to comparatively severe limitations and inconvenience. I recall seeing a bus driver who had last been examined five years previously. His prescription approximated to R and L + 1.00DS with a + 1.25DS reading addition. His distance refraction had increased by about 1.50 dioptres, so that his original reading prescription was now practically correct for distance. He was wearing an old pair of 22 mm round segment bifocals, and had developed the habit of tilting his head back and looking through the reading portion in order to see to drive his bus! Astonishingly, the only symptom he mentioned when he came for re-examination was of difficulty in reading.

18.7   Varifocals

Special difficulties can arise with varifocals. It can happen that the prescription is too weak, and the patient has got into the habit of tilting the head back, thus using some part of the transitional zone for distance vision. If he or she continues to do this when the lenses have been updated, there will be a complaint that vision is blurred outdoors. For the same reason you may have found an increase in plus after performing refraction, which you feel sure will improve the acuity in comparison with the old prescription, but when you attempt to demonstrate this the patient insists there is no difference.

My dispenser recently showed me a new pair of varifocal spectacles that he had just checked, when he had discovered that although the powers were 'correct', both lenses had been cut from a blank intended for the left eye. Yet they bore the manufacturer's markings exactly as would have been placed on a properly matched pair. If the distance portion only had been checked, and the marked reading additions accepted as correct, it would have presented a nice problem for the prescriber to solve at some later date. This is a good example of just one of the multifarious possibilities that have to be taken into account when dealing with 'intolerance' or 'grief' cases. It must be emphasized, incidentally, that this section cannot attempt to give a comprehensive account of all such possibilities; the main object is to provide guidance by furnishing a wide selection of problems actually encountered in practice.

Incidentally it is wise to ask to see the old spectacles even with a regular patient. Not infrequently it will be found (especially with aged patients who have numerous pairs) that they are wearing the wrong ones; the lenses may be so badly scratched or the frames in such poor condition that they will need to be replaced whether or not there is any difference in the prescription.

18.8   The patient's symptoms

Case history taking, where refraction is concerned, should have elicited the patient's reasons for coming for examination, especially in regard to leisure or occupational requirements. (Part 1 has dealt with the main questions to be asked for the eye examination itself). A useful opening question is 'Have you come just for a routine check, or are you having some particular difficulty in seeing?' *It is most important to remember what the patient gives as his reason for seeking advice.* Perhaps he says he only wants new reading glasses, for instance, but after performing the refraction you consider that a distance pair should be a higher priority.

By all means explain this to him, heavily emphasising the need if he cannot achieve the legal standard for driving unless he wears spectacles for this purpose. But don't try to dissuade him from what he knows his requirements are. The student is sometimes amazed when he first encounters people with 6/18 vision or worse, but who maintain that they can see perfectly clearly for distance, and appear not the slightest bit impressed when he demonstrates that they can achieve 6/6 with correction. There is usually nothing at all mysterious in this attitude. It is either due to vanity – they don't want to be seen wearing glasses; or economy – they are not prepared to go to the expense of a second pair. If vanity is the only reason, however, distance spectacles will often be accepted if it is explained that they will greatly enhance the clarity of television programmes and that they do not have to wear them outdoors unless they wish to.

Bear in mind that descriptions of symptoms vary extremely widely, partly because they are by their very nature subjective. The temperament and status of the individual are relevant; the man with a calamitous or severely deprived background, for instance, may experience exactly the same symptoms as a more prosperous contemporary, without perceiving them as so serious or distressing. Remember also that there is occasionally an exceedingly simple solution for what looks like a dramatic visual problem, as the next two examples illustrate.

Mistaken identity

This patient had attended regularly in the past for routine checks; her corrected acuity was good, and she was not in the least inclined to complain. She had recently been in hospital for a major operation, but when she returned home, she found she was unable to see with her glasses. Understandably, she thought that her sight must have suffered as a result of her illness, and was very worried. Looking at her old frame, it was realized that it was not of a type we had supplied, though it did resemble the original pair. On checking the lens powers, it was discovered that they were not her glasses at all; they must have inadvertently been exchanged for those belonging to the patient in the next bed while she was in hospital. She was immediately relieved and delighted to find that with the correct lenses her sight was unimpaired, and that there had actually been very little change in her prescription.

Confusion

A very irate middle-aged woman stormed into the consulting room, complaining noisily that both her pairs of glasses, supplied only a fortnight before, were 'completely useless'. She only calmed down when she was assured that we did not want to have dissatisfied patients, and that whatever the problem was, it would be put right. There is no point in losing your temper with such persons; after all, the lenses *might* indeed have been wrong, at worst, she could conceivably have been handed out spectacles intended for somebody else – and people do not usually get as worked up as this unless they really believe that they have a genuine complaint.

The first step, therefore, was to check the lenses without getting involved in any argument. They were, it transpired, quite correct, but she had confused the distance with the reading pair, and had become so annoyed that she had failed to notice that when used at the proper distance they were excellent. When this was explained to her, patiently and without annoyance, she burst into tears and apologized profusely.

An aggressive response in a case like this would have been totally inappropriate. She was not an unpleasant person at all; her exaggerated reaction was due to her excitable temperament and her conviction that she had paid out money she could ill afford without deriving any benefit.

18.9   Procedure for investigating complaints

You will frequently have to deal with a patient who is complaining about his spectacles – whether supplied by yourself or by somebody else. These complaints are often vague and not to the point; he insists they are uncomfortable but fails to provide clear reasons for his dissatisfaction. One therefore needs to be aware of the major possible sources of trouble, and to develop a method for resolving these cases.

The following list of points to be checked or considered, roughly in order of their importance, may be helpful; it cannot be comprehensive, because from time to time one encounters unusual or bizarre difficulties that could not possibly have been anticipated. Keep in mind, however, that so far as is possible *you should avoid making any comments before you have identified the problem.*

Fitting

Are the sides too long/short/wrongly angled/not filed out sufficiently/need bowing? Are the lashes touching? Is the frame level? Does the bridge fit properly?

Check prescription

(Remember BVP may be relevant.) Check horizontal centring, also vertical where necessary. Any flaws or scratches on lenses?

Compare old prescription and fitting

Is the degree of change made disconcerting to the patient?

Reading addition

Is it appropriate for habitual reading or work distance? Is the older pair preferred for intermediate distances because it gives a longer range? Is it balanced R and L?

Is the visual acuity as good as that recorded?

Is it in fact better with the previous pair? If visual acuity is for some reason worse in one eye, has it been explained to the patient that this is the best that can be done? Is there any disturbance of binocular vision?

Multifocals

Check segment height, depth, and inset. Is it that the type of lens supplied is different (e.g. flat top instead of round) and that this is disconcerting to the patient? Special attention to varifocals – monocular acuity may improve with tilt or turn of head if centring is inaccurate.

Is weight a cause of discomfort?

Is the thickness excessive? Are the lenses properly matched for thickness (allowing, of course, for anisometropic differences)?

'Tilting' effects

Usually associated with changes in astigmatic correction. Check axes carefully. If correct, but appreciably different from the previous prescription this symptom is probably only transient.

Other problems

'Jack-in-the-box' phenomenon with high plus powers; Aniseikonic effects, associated perhaps with anisometropic prescriptions. Change of base curves may explain why a patient has difficulty adjusting to a spare, 'matching' pair of lenses.

Possible changes

Beware of possible changes which could have arisen since the date of test. These are relatively rare, but the writer has seen a considerable number of such cases, where lesions such as retinal haemorrhages, detachment, iritis, or field defects have occurred within days or weeks of examination – occasionally even before the spectacles have been supplied!

Ulterior motives

The complainants who have an ulterior motive are more difficult to cope with, (fortunately they are not encountered very often). The explanation may be very simple, but extremely difficult to uncover. The patient may have seen some other item on which he wishes to lavish expenditure, and hopes that by making enough fuss he will be able to get money back for this purpose; or he may have regretted his choice of spectacles and is trying to get out of his commitment in order to re-purchase elsewhere.

Neurotic patients

Last, and most difficult of all, are the neurotics, and the psychologically disorientated patients who either invent symptoms for no reason whatsoever, or want to show the professional man that he is not *that* clever; no positive cause for their complaints can be found, or as soon as one complaint is countered a new objection is raised.

I recall encountering one such person early in my experience whose symptoms puzzled me so much that I telephoned his GP for advice. 'It's no fault of yours', he reassured me. 'I could have told you even before you started your test that the spectacles weren't going to be any good. Nothing is ever right for this patient'. The moral is obvious. If you can recognize this type of individual (and with experience together with perceptivity in case history taking you often can), don't undertake dispensing unless it is absolutely necessary.

Chapter 19
Patients' Records

19.1   Examples of the value of retinoscopy as an aid to refraction

Case 1   Male, aged 26

This young man had been seen only 18 months before, when visual acuity with lenses was R 6/5, L 6/6. He had since been affected with bilateral optic neuritis. As a result, he was unable to recognize any of the numbers in the Ishihara book apart from the first test plate; a central scotoma was present in each eye, more extensively in the left, and visual acuity was so severely affected that ordinary subjective refraction could not be relied upon. Retinoscopy gave:

$$R \; -3.75/-1.00 \times 95$$
$$L \; -3.75/-1.00 \times 85$$

This was very similar to the prescription in his own spectacles, with which he could read only R 6/18, L 6/60 (by eccentric fixation). Modifications subjectively made no difference. Retinoscopy provided confirmation that the poor acuity was not due to incorrect assessment of the refractive error.

Case 2   Female, aged 44

A similar case, with bilateral optic atrophy was seen in which the acuities were only R 3/60, L 1/60. Retinoscopy showed that there was virtually no refractive error present, so that this could be eliminated as a factor in the assessment of her visual problems.

Case 3   Female, aged 60

This lady was completely illiterate, but required glasses for sewing and mending. Retinoscopy provided a rapid measure of her quite considerable distance refractive error, and the appropriate prescription for close work could then be ascertained with ease. Incidentally, it is useful to have a book of reading charts that includes a needle and thread, allowing a practical demonstration of the advantage of spectacles in cases like this.

166

Case 4   Female, aged 36

This patient had been told for many years that her left eye was severely defective, and had accepted that she could only see the top few lines on the test chart with it. She was wearing:

> R – 2.00 cyl × 85
> L – 1.00/ – 3.00 × 95

As soon as retinoscopy was attempted, it was evident that the left prescription was incorrect – the true cylinder was approximately – 4.00 cyl at 110. After refining this by subjective refraction the final result was:

> L – 1.25/ – 4.00 × 107½ 6/12 +

The acuity tended to fluctuate during refraction, but she expressed great surprise at the improvement. She said that vision binocularly was noticeably more comfortable, although the R acuity was considerably better at 6/5. When seen again, several years later, the L refraction was still about the same but the acuity had improved to a steady 6/9 + .

Case 5   Female, aged 36

This was a similar case, a lady of the same age who had not been carefully refracted because one eye was assumed to have always been very defective. She had a low degree L oblique convergent strabismus. Her present spectacles were:

> R + 1.75/ – 3.75 × 175
> L + 2.00/ – 2.75 × 15

Retinoscopy showed a small increase in the R astigmatic power, but the left was quite different. Because of the strabismus, the R eyes was occluded and the L refracted by the dynamic method, which revealed that the correct cylinder was in the region of 6.00 dioptres. This was confirmed subjectively, the final prescription being:

> R + 1.75/ – 4.25 × 175 6/6 +
> L – 0.25/6.00 × 10 6/12

Although she did not get normal binocular vision, she much preferred the change with the L lens, and has returned many times for rechecking and replacement spectacles. In such cases, if the full correction can be worn with comfort, it should be given. In the unfortunate event of some disaster befalling the good eye, the other will then respond more readily to the demands placed upon it. At the same time, it must be mentioned that some people are quite unable to wear a full prescription comfortably, especially if there is appreciable anisometropia, and careful consideration has to be given to find the best compromise.

Case 6   Male, aged 76

This man had just lost his distance spectacles, and came in for a recheck of his refraction prior to having them replaced. He had not been seen in the practice before and the old *reading* prescription was:

R + 5.75/ – 0.50 × 75
L + 5.75/ – 0.50 × 125

Immediately retinoscopy was commenced, it was evident that the cylinders had been set incorrectly, or that their axes had altered very greatly, because the new settings were found to be R 110 degrees, L 75 degrees. Wearing the retinoscopy correction and without any subjective modifications being made at this stage, he was able to read R and L 6/6. At this point I focimetered the old spectacles myself, in case they had been incorrectly measured by the dispenser. But they were correct, which meant that the patient should be encouraged to have both pairs replaced. It will be realized that if the pair which were broken had also been set at the wrong axes (which was most probable) he would be likely to experience greater difficulty if he had this put right, but had the axes reversed each time he changed to his reading glasses.

Differences like this are sometimes found because a practitioner has tested the patient's left eye first, but inadvertently written the prescription down for the right eye. If one eye is known to be more defective, for instance, it is sometimes better to deal with it first, in case the patient memorizes the letters, but it is obviously necessary to take care in committing the details to the record card.

Case 7   Male, aged 40

This patient was mentally defective, and had a complete L cataract. He was unable to recognize any letters or figures, and could not trace the lines on the Ishihara plates. However, his GP had requested that his refraction should be checked, and also wished to know if the IOP was normal.

Sheridan-Gardiner tests gave a poor 6/9 for the right eye. It was fortunately easy to perform retinoscopy, which revealed practically no refractive error. The IOP was found to be normal.

Case 8   Female, aged 68

The spectacles worn were said to have never been comfortable, either for distance or reading. The prescription was:

R + 1.25/ – 0.25 × 100
L + 1.75/ – 1.00 × 105   Add + 2.25 reading

Retinoscopy indicated slightly higher plus in the right eye than the left, but the refraction initially found was:

R $+1.75/-1.50 \times 100$ 6/6 +
L $+1.75/-1.25 \times 105$ 6/6 +

In view of the retinoscopy findings attempts were made to further relax accommodation by 'plussing-up' and binocular refraction. After a few minutes the right eye accepted a further $+0.25$. Confirmation that this was in fact correct was given by binocular balance being also present at the reading distance with the same reading addition for each eye.

Case 9 Female, aged 50

Delay in relaxation of accommodation is more commonly found in younger patients, but this case (as also in the above) shows that one must be prepared for this possibility in older people. The old spectacles were:

R $+1.50/-0.25 \times 115$ 6/5
L $+1.50/-0.25 \times 65$ 6/5   (Add $+1.25$ reading)

She complained of persistent vague discomfort with these, for both distance and reading. In this case, retinoscopy indicated definitely higher plus in the left eye than the right. Subjective refraction:

R 6/12 + $+1.25/-0.25 \times 110$ 6/5
L 6/12 $+1.50/-0.25 \times 45$ 6/5

As this small difference seemed to be less than retinoscopy had indicated binocular additions were tried, as well as the effect of 'plussing-up' one eye while rechecking the refraction of the other.

Another useful aid to relaxation of accommodation, which was tried in this instance, is to stimulate positive relative convergence by putting 6^Δ base out before one eye, while the patient reads the smallest letters manageable on the distance chart. If diplopia occurs, this will often disappear if the patient is asked to look at a near object and then revert to the distance target. Provided single vision is maintained, convergence is being exercised in excess of accommodation. When the prism is removed, it will often be found that the accommodation relaxes further, so that a monocular or binocular addition will be accepted. Applied in this case, it revealed that the full L sphere should have been $+1.75$. This was again confirmed by near binocular balance being achieved with equal reading additions of R and L $+1.25$DS.

It will be realized that had this additional plus acceptance not been uncovered, there would have been no real justification to alter her existing prescription.

Case 10   Male, aged 22   Retinoscopy and latent hypermetropia

This was a foreign student who had never been refracted before. His complaint was of tiredness after reading, and persistent blurring with his left eye. Retinoscopy showed quite a high error to be present:

Ret. R + 6.00DS   L + 7.00/ − 0.50 × H

He had a low degree variable L convergent strabismus. Refraction was difficult due to fluctuating vision as a result of ciliary cramp:

R 6/12 + 3.00DS 6/12 +
L 6/36 + 4.00DS 6/18
11$^\triangle$Esophoria   Ortho. V distance

Any increase in plus sphere produced an immediate complaint of blurring, so he was given the above prescription as the best compromise until the ciliary cramp began to subside. I would not prescribe the full theoretical prescription in a case like this, as it simply would not have been worn, especially as there was very little improvement in distance acuity even with the reduced powers as above.

19.2   Subjective refraction

Case 11   Female, aged 41   Insufficient plus and fan charts

This patient said she had suffered with headaches and ocular discomfort for several years past. She had previously been tested about a year ago, when she had been told there was no change in the prescription, and her glasses were not altered. She was wearing:

R − 1.00DS (6/12 +)
L − 1.00/ − 0.25 × 50 (6/9 +)

Retinoscopy indicated very definite horizontal cylinders, and subjective refraction was as anticipated:

R − 0.50/ − 1.00 × 170 6/6 +
L − 0.50/ − 0.50 ×   5 6/6 +

One can only speculate as to why she had been checked and the discrepancy not found, but the most likely explanation is that the previous prescriber had started off with too much minus, so that she was unable to distinguish the blacker lines on the fan chart with any certainty. The reader may well question the assumption that she had been tested with the fan and blocks, but if cross-cylinders were used the results could not have become confused in this way. She was so relieved when the new prescription was tried out, that it was considered of interest to recheck her vision with the original prescription. The result (shown in brackets above) was worse than expected, and it was no wonder that she had had so much discomfort.

Case 12   Female, aged 65   Fan and block test inapplicable here

There were extensive lens changes present, especially with the right eye, and a satisfactory retinoscopy could not be performed. She had been wearing the following prescription during the previous two years:

R $+1.75/-2.00 \times 165$
L $+1.50/-1.00 \times 45$

She made no particular complaint about her vision, and had come for a routine check. The exact prescription was very different:

R $+1.50/-1.50 \times 75$ 6/12 +
L $+1.50/-1.00 \times 25$ 6/9 +

The refraction was assessed by cross-cylinders and turning the lenses to confirm that the best position had been found. She was unable to distinguish any real difference with the fan and blocks, and said that they looked much the same to her whether the R cylinder was set at 165 degrees or 75 degrees. However, so far as visual acuity was concerned, there was a great difference – she could only see 6/24 with the axis at 165.

Case 13   Female, aged 52   Insufficient plus sphere component

This case was the subject of an Ophthalmic Services Committee investigation. The patient complained that an extremely cursory test had been performed — allegedly taking only five minutes, following which the following prescription was issued:

R $+0.50$DS
L $+0.50$DS   Add $+2.00$ reading

Dissatisfied, the patient attended another practitioner, when a completely different result was found:

R $+1.50/-0.50 \times 15$ 6/5
L $+1.75/-0.75 \times 180$ 6/5   Add $+1.75$ reading

Arrangements were made for the patient to be examined independently by a third party, who found the stronger prescription correct – his correction varied by only about 0.25 and a small change in axis direction. This case highlights several points. First, if a reasonable retinoscopy had been carried out on the first occasion, it is unlikely that an error of this dimension could possibly have been made.

Secondly, if the sphere is this far out, it is just not possible to assess the astigmatic element. And thirdly, the reading addition could not have been properly checked because it was quite insufficient. One other point which could be mentioned is that if the reading addition found looks rather high for the age of the patient concerned, it is wise to check back on the distance refraction, and to see if a distance binocular addition is acceptable.

Case 14   Male, aged 64   Too much plus affecting cross cyl result

With this patient, the correct prescription eventually found was:

R – 0.50/ – 0.50 × 10   6/5
L – 0.50 cyl × 170   6/6 +

Initially, the L cylinder axis came out at 100, judging from his replies in the cross-cyl test. It was realized that this must be wrong, partly because of the retinoscopy results, and also because the visual acuity was not very good and tended to vary. It was presently discovered that the basic sphere for the left eye had been overestimated from the start, and cross-cylinder checking was attempted with + 0.50 or + 0.75DS in the trial frame. The result of this would have been that in one position the cross cylinder focused one meridian practically on the retina; in the other, the two meridians coincided, but were too far forward for this to be recognized as clearer.

The mistake was soon realized, of course, as soon as the sphere was reduced in the interest of best vision, and the cross-cyl test repeated. Discrepancies due to incorrect sphere power are much more likely to occur in fan and block testing than with the cross-cylinder, incidentally; in the illustration just given the error would have been much less likely if the cylinder power had been other than 0.50DC.

Case 15   Female, aged 15   Degree of tolerance acceptable

Many of the cases described are cautionary tales indicating the care necessary for accurate refraction. A small error in sphere, cylinder, or axis, or the omission of a weak prism, will often result in patient dissatisfaction of a surprisingly high order, apart from the trouble and expense involved in trying to put things right. Yet occasionally one encounters patients wearing completely wrong prescriptions without complaint. In the instance under discussion, the girl had brought her spectacles in for a minor repair, when it was noticed that the lenses had somehow been transposed left for right. They were a PRO shape and could therefore be changed over in this way. The prescription was:

R $- 3.50/ - 3.50 \times 30$
L $- 3.50/ - 3.00 \times 150$

As she had made no complaint of difficulty in seeing, the lenses were quickly changed over and the spectacles handed back without comment. Astonishingly, there was simply no reaction. Asked if she noticed any difference, she simply replied, 'Oh, they're all right'. If any reader does not realize how extraordinary this is, he should look through a $- 3.00$D cyl crossed with a $+ 3.00$D cyl at 60 degrees, and then turn them so that their axes are coincident. That is the amount of difference the patient was expected to notice in this case!

Case 16   Male, aged 68   Tolerance and depth of focus

This was another case of tolerance to incorrect prescriptions, but much more understandable. He had been prescribed the following prescription about two years before:

R $+ 1.75/ - 1.00 \times 80$
L $+ 2.00/ - 1.00 \times 77\frac{1}{2}$ Add $+ 2.50$ reading

While he was in India, he asked to have a spare pair made up. He was satisfied with these, but the prescription was:

R $+ 1.25$DS (6/9)
L $+ 1.25$DS (6/12)   Add $+ 2.25$ reading

He had evidently been given the nearest spheres possible from stock! Refracting him now, the following result was found:

R $+ 2.00/ - 0.75 \times 65$ 6/6
L $+ 1.75/ - 0.75 \times 120$ 6/6   Add $+ 2.50$ reading

In spite of the difference in axis of the L cylinder, he said he did not really notice a great deal of difference with any of them. However, he had minute, almost pin-point pupils, which would have given him an increased depth of focus and made the discrepancies less noticeable. Even so, it will be noted that the *measured* visual acuity, with the latest pair of spheres, was considerably worse than with the latest correction found.

Cases in which orthodox subjective methods were inapplicable

Case 17   Male, aged 73

This patient had had keratitis as a child of nine. As a result there was deep old corneal scarring and central hazing, more marked in the right eye. Retinoscopy was consequently quite impossible, and there was no hope of his recognizing any difference on the fan test. Cross cylinders provided some help, but were only a rough guide. He was wearing:

R $-0.50/-0.50 \times 90$
L $+1.50/-0.50 \times 90$ Add $+3.00$ R, $+2.50$ L reading

How does one start with a case like this? The first step was to see if the acuity obtained with his old lenses would improve with the pinhole disc. This was found to be the case, indicating that some radical change was required. The empirical method adopted here was to assess the maximum plus which was acceptable without increasing the distance blur, and then to increase this by $+0.50$ DS (as one would for testing with a fan chart). Next a cylinder of appreciable power – in this instance a -2.00 D cyl – was inserted at axis vertical. The reason for starting off with a vertical axis was because of the patient's age. So-called 'with-the-rule' astigmatism (minus axis horizontal) predominates in children and the younger age groups; 'against-the-rule' (minus axis vertical) is usual in older persons. By a combination of cross-cylinder technique and turning the cylinder in the trial frame by hand, a 'best axis' was determined. The next step was to refine the power, and in this case visual acuity improved as the cylinder was increased, and then to modify the spherical element. The final result obtained was:

R 6/36 $+1.25/-3.50 \times 105$ 6/15
L 6/24 $+4.25/-2.50 \times 85$ 6/9 –   Add $+2.50$ reading

The patient was vastly impressed with the improvement in his vision, and it was deplorable that a better result had not been achieved with his previous test. There is nothing magical about discovering the full prescription in cases like this, only a combination of logic and patience. This example of course provides another illustration for the need to put in sufficient plus sphere to begin with, whether for fan and block or empirical methods of testing. The previous examiner had evidently started off with insufficient plus, and would in consequence never arrive at the correct astigmatic element.

Case 18   Male, aged 38   Very high astigmatic element

This was another case in which vision was affected – even more severely – by corneal scarring and distortion. The refraction seemed to change unpredictably with the slightest shift of view or head tilt. The old prescription was:

R $+4.00/-9.50 \times 90$
L $+1.00/-3.00 \times 100$

It was again only possible to attempt refraction by trying in lenses and turning the cylinders to obtain the best vision possible. Using a + 1.00 cross cylinder (e.g. a + 1.00/ − 2.00c) he was able to perceive sufficient difference, some of the time, for this to be of some help. The correction eventually found was:

R + 1.00/ − 10.00 × 95 6/12 +
L + 5.00/ − 8.00 × 95 6/36

The standard achieved with the right eye was much better than to be expected with such a high power, but it was not maintained easily and the acuity tended to fade off after a short time. Note the extraordinary difference in sphere powers obtained for the new prescription. Nevertheless, when his visual acuity with the old prescription was checked for comparison (always a wise procedure, this; in these difficult cases one's best guesses may be wrong!) he was still able to read nearly 6/15 with the right eye.

He was asked to report back after a few weeks to see if he found much benefit from the change. He said that he did, but was still not particularly comfortable. He tended to revert to his old pair for close work, probably because the higher sphere acted as a reading addition. He had found another practitioner who was proposing to fit him with contact lenses, which should theoretically be better by filling in some of the corneal irregularities with the tear film, provided that rotation of the lenses could be minimized.

Case 19   Female, aged 62   Stenopaeic slit refraction

This was another case of old bilateral corneal scarring, which was so bad with her left eye that it had always been regarded as practically blind. The right eye could be refracted normally, using the cross-cylinder, but the L was much more of a problem. The old prescription was:

R + 2.50/ − 2.50 × 30
L + 1.00DS

It was quite impossible to attempt retinoscopy on the left eye, but keratometry revealed some irregular astigmatism, and indicated a minus axis approximately along the 20 degree meridian. Empirical testing was not very fruitful, but the pinhole disc had shown that it should be possible to make some improvement. It was therefore decided to perform stenopaeic slit refraction. This entailed setting the slit initially along the 20-degree meridian, and tilting it slightly to the position the patient thought was clearest. This meridian was then refracted, using spheres. Next the slit was rotated 90 degrees and refraction with spheres repeated in this meridian. When the resultant sphero-cylindrical combination was worked out and put into the trial frame, some improvement was found, which was then fined off by minor adjustments to the prescription. The final results were:

R 6/24 + 2.75/ − 3.25 × 30 6/9
L 6/60 + 2.25/ − 2.00 × 12½ 6/24

The improvement achieved was not marvellous, but was of course very much better than with the + 1.00DS previously worn. It was certainly worthwhile making this alteration because there was virtually no ocular muscle imbalance and she did get binocular vision.

Case 20   Male, aged 19   Exceptionally difficult refraction case

This young man had had bilateral operations for congenital cataract which had not been outstandingly successful. There was irregular 'after-cataract' in both eyes, and the L had a variable divergent strabismus. The R pupil area was obscured by filmy tissue except for a small 'window' in its upper nasal aspect, so retinoscopy was out of the question. He was wearing bifocals prescribed by a very able and experienced practitioner:

R + 3.50DS
L + 4.25/ − 2.25 × 120   Add + 3.00 reading

I made the refraction:

R 6/15 + 3.25/ − 0.75 × 90 6/12 partly
L 6/24 + 4.25/ − 0.75 × 100 6/15

He was referred to an ophthalmic surgeon before considering dispensing, who prescribed 1/8th% atropine to produce some enlargement of the pupils, and mentioned that if vision was not satisfactory he proposed to perform a further capsulotomy. His prescription was:

R + 2.50/ − 1.00 × 30
L + 2.50/ − 2.50 × 120

It may seem incredible that three different experienced people could arrive at such widely differing results within a short space of time. It would be very difficult to say whether one was right and the others were wrong, because the patient obtained just about the same visual acuity with each of the three prescriptions. Fortunately such cases are extremely rare, and I would class it among the most difficult refractive problems I have encountered.

Impracticability of prescribing in anisometropia

Case 21   Male, aged 60

This patient had suffered damage to his right eye as a result of exposure to a sunlamp as a child. There was an old iritic adhesion (posterior synechia) at the upper aspect of the pupil, and atrophic changes surrounding the disc. He said that his right eye had never been 'fully examined', because it had been permanently damaged. Nevertheless he had always worried in case some accident should befall his good eye. The prescription worn was:

R $- 5.50/ - 1.75 \times 175$
L $- 2.25/ - 0.25 \times 10$

The right eye tended to diverge on cover test – a latent divergent strabismus. Retinoscopy was attempted, but the image was too dim to interpret with the right eye. This often gives a hint that there may be a high minus refractive error, which was confirmed subjectively. When a $- 10.00DS$ was put in, he was very surprised at the improvement, and vision was then good enough to go ahead with normal cross-cylinder refraction. The correct prescription was found to be:

R $- 10.50/ - 2.50 \times 115$ 6/9 partly
L $- 1.25/ - 0.25 \; \times 80$ 6/5

In anisometropia of this degree it is not feasible to attempt bilateral correction. However, if a reduced prescription is given the cylinder should be set at the correct axis. The reduction made, moreover, should be drastic enough to avoid producing binocular confusion. It was decided in this case to give $- 5.00/ - 2.00 \times 115$ for the right eye. The patient was greatly relieved to learn that his defective eye could achieve reasonably good vision if the need ever arrived.

Case 22   Female, aged 60   Circumspection in making drastic changes

This case was the subject of a complaint to the Ophthalmic Investigation Committee. The prescription worn by the patient when she was examined by the practitioner concerned, was:

R $- 16.50/ - 2.25 \times 85$ $1\frac{1}{2}^{\Delta}$ base down 6/9 partly
L $- 18.00/ - 3.25 \times 85$ $1\frac{1}{2}^{\Delta}$ base up 6/18

The correction he found on this occasion was very different:

R $- 19.00/ - 2.25 \times 85$ 6/18
L $- 20.50/ - 4.50 \times 85$ 6/18

The full prescription was dispensed, and the patient was told that she could wear her old distance pair for reading. Unfortunately, she was quite unable to get on with this increased prescription, and complained of giddiness, tilting effects, and other symptoms. She returned to the prescriber, who assured her that she would get used to them, but she was still very unhappy, and took the matter further.

An ophthalmic surgeon saw her later, who stated that although objectively she did not appear to be over-corrected, subjectively she found the new prescription quite intolerable. He added that very short-sighted people will often not tolerate the full prescription, and continued, 'With her old glasses she had slight esophoria without any symptoms, but with the new ones she had definite small degree alternating convergent squint with double vision.'

This case could have been resolved much more easily but for the fact that the practitioner could not accept that he had made an error in prescribing. The fact that the actual powers prescribed may have been correct did not necessarily mean that they would be wearable. One should always be very circumspect in regard to making changes of this magnitude, especially in an elderly patient. The other interesting aspect of this problem was the induced diplopia. It was evident that with her old, weak prescription, she was using virtually no accommodation when viewing objects at intermediate or near distances. The sudden increase in concave power, however, provided a stimulus to convergence for which she was unprepared, precipitating the diplopia.

There is always a danger for us all in prescribing to permit theoretical considerations to over-ride practical ones. It is wise to remember Dr Laurence Peter's dictum: 'The patient *knows* that he is suffering, whether the physician will admit it or not'.

Case 23   Male, aged 60   Refraction with severe field restriction

This patient had suffered with retinitis pigmentosa for many years, and came to see if any improvement could be made in his vision. He was carrying a white stick, but it transpired that it was not solely to indicate that he was virtually blind. When directed to the letter chart, he asked me to point his stick to it, so that he could sight along it and find out where it was. Aiming it was not so easy as might be imagined, and he tended to 'lose' the chart occasionally, and needed to be realigned. With a weak convex prescription he was able to read almost R and L 6/6, but his field was so small that it did not encompass the whole 6/6 line. He had tubular fields of about 1 degree, which must have been much more of a handicap than central field loss with peripheral retention.

Case 24   Female, aged 68   Anomalous duochrome results

Generally speaking, duochrome tests are extemely accurate and repeatable; many patients are sensitive to differences of a fraction of a dioptre. On the other hand, if too much reliance is placed on these tests misleading results can occur. In the case under discussion, the prescription found, which gave exact binocular balance, with 0.25 red dominance on each side, was:

> R 6/36 + 2.00/ − 0.50 × 45 6/5
> L 6/18 + 2.00/ − 0.50 × 125 6/5   Add + 2.25 reading

The only difference between this and her old prescription was that the previous L sphere had been 1.75 instead of 2.00. It did not seem worth altering her spectacles for this small amount, but as she had complained of slight ocular discomfort attempts were made to see if a binocular addition could be accepted. There was no appreciable muscle balance defect. To verify the difference, the duochrome test was repeated with her wearing the old spectacles. Surprisingly, she still reported exact balance, and there was still 0.25 red dominance with each eye. For near work, there was precise balance of accommodation with her old lenses, but slight preference to the left eye with the extra 0.25 put on. Quite obviously there was no intention of changing her lenses, but the example highlights the point that even with the most careful assessment of the binocular balance, small errors or differences can still occur. The probable reason is that the patient is just not so fussy about what we are aiming to achieve as she should be.

Case 25   Male, aged 64   Unilateral insensitivity to duochrome tests

This patient had a L divergent strabismus, but tended to alternate. He was quite highly myopic:

> R − 14.50/ − 3.00 × 22½ 6/9 +
> L − 15.00/ − 3.50 × 155 6/12 +   Add + 3.00 reading

With bichromatic tests persistent red dominance was obtained with his right eye. He still maintained that the circles were clearer on the red with a − 1.25 increase in sphere. If any more minus was added, he said both sets of circles were blurred. With his left eye, although it did not achieve such good acuity, the tests were consistent and reasonably precise and an 0.37 minus sphere turned him over from red dominance to green. Because of the squint, it was no good attempting to blur one eye up with more plus, while checking the other. The decision on the final sphere for the right eye had to be judged by the minimum minus which gave the best acuity. This, after all, is how it always used to be done before bichromatic tests became the norm, but when one has become fully accustomed to these tests, one does not feel so confident without them.

Case 26   Female, aged 40   Bilateral insensitivity to duochrome tests

This was really a perfectly easy and straightforward case of refraction. There was no complaint of visual difficulty, and she was nearly emmetropic:

> R + 0.25DS 6/5
> L + 0.50/ – 0.25 × 80 6/5 Orthophoric V and H Distance

After determining the refraction, one attempts to ensure that the correct sphere element has been ascertained by utilizing the bichromatic type tests, but in this instance it was just not possible to produce green dominance at all. She was quite positive that the circles were clearer on the red background even with the addition of – 1.00s, either monocularly or binocularly. Yet with these additional lenses she said that the letters were less clear. Such results are not all that unusual; sometimes they are due to the fact that the patient is not paying full attention to what is required, but at other times it presumably means that the usual chromatic aberration present in the ocular optical system is absent or lacking.

Even when the normal amount of chromatism is present, bichromatic tests are not very good for ascertaining the best vision sphere where there are high cylinders or poor visual acuity, because they are rarely sensitive enough in such cases.

Unusual changes in refraction

Case 27   Male, aged 58   Diabetic refractive changes (not reversing)

This patient's refraction had not altered much over a considerable period. At the time of his last test, early lens changes had been noted, and the refraction was:

> R 6/36 – 1.25 cyl × 100 6/6
> L 6/36 + 0.25/ × – 2.25 × 45 6/6

Now, two years later, the lens changes had advanced somewhat, and the refraction had altered to:

> R 6/60 – 2.00/ – 1.25 × 95 6/12 +
> L 6/60 – 1.75/ – 2.50 × 55 6/12 +

One might well ask why he had not presented himself earlier, as the corrected vision was much worse now, with the old lenses. Marked changes like this, usually in the myopic direction and bi-lateral, are highly suspicious of diabetes. Questioning revealed that his mother, paternal grandfather, and two sisters, were all diabetic. After referral it was found that he was similarly affected. He was put on dieting and treatment but even after satisfactory stabilization some months later the refractive changes had not reversed.

Case 28   Male, aged 47   Diabetic refractive changes (reversing)

This patient had never been examined and had not worn glasses before, and until very recently had not experienced any difficulty in seeing. He now found his distance vision appreciably blurred. The refraction indicated an appreciable degree of myopia, which could not have been present before because his work demanded a good standard of vision:

$$R \; 6/15 \; -1.75/-0.75 \times 180 \; 6/6+$$
$$L \; 6/24 \; -1.75/-0.50 \times 180 \; 6/6+$$

The noticeably poorer VA in the left eye suggested that this eye required a higher prescription – one has to watch for pointers like this. But in fact the prescription found balanced perfectly on binocular tests. It transpired that he had recently had symptoms of excessive thirst, and on referral diabetes was confirmed. Four months later, after treatment and stabilization, he returned for a further check on his refraction:

$$R \; 6/6 \; -0.75 \; \text{cyl} \times 10 \; 6/5$$
$$L \; 6/6 \; -0.25/-0.50 \times 180 \; 6/5$$

This is more typical of a recently diagnosed diabetic case, where the increase in myopia reverses after treatment. For this reason, it is advisable never to dispense spectacles for these patients until stabilization has been obtained.

Case 29   Male, aged 40   Unaccountable changes in refraction

Where sudden changes in refraction occur, it is wise to be cautious before making alterations. This was a regular patient, whose prescription had never varied much in the past. He was wearing:

$$R \; +0.75/-0.75 \times 175 \; 6/5$$
$$L \; +0.50/-0.50 \times 15 \; \; 6/5$$

He came now because his distance sight seemed to have suddenly altered. The prescription now was:

$$R \; +1.50 \; (\text{or} \; 1.75)/-0.75 \times 175 \; 6/5$$
$$L \; +1.25/-0.75 \times 10 \; 6/5$$

There were no significant ophthalmoscopic signs, but he was referred for medical investigations, which proved negative. However, he returned again after a month, when the prescription had reverted almost to the original. He has been refracted on a number of occasions since, but no appreciable further changes in distance refraction have occurred.

Case 30   Female, aged 31   Inexplicable reversing refractive changes

In this instance the change was unilateral, more marked, and lasted for a longer period of time. The original refraction was:

> R + 2.50/ – 1.00 × 55 6/5
> L + 2.50/ – 0.50 × 125 6/5

The patient suddenly noticed that her vision was more blurred in her left eye when the glasses were worn, and lost little time in coming for advice. On this visit, only nine months later, the prescription had altered to:

> R 6/9 + 2.50/ – 0.50 × 70 6/5
> L 6/9 + 0.75/ – 0.75 × 115 6/9

Again no abnormality could be detected, though the L corrected acuity was down. She was referred, and seen by a consultant the next day, but he was unable to account for the change. She returned for re-checking a few weeks later. This time refraction was performed under cycloplegia, but the difference of nearly two dioptres between the two eyes was confirmed. However, the L acuity had now returned to nearly 6/5 again. She was not at all comfortable with the prescription, of course, but one naturally hesitates to make an alteration of this dimension. After a further week with no change, therefore, a new pair were dispensed, which proved quite satisfactory for about three months, when she came in again to announce a sudden change in her vision.

The refraction of the left eye had now reverted to almost exactly what it was in the first place. The L lens was therefore altered once more, but the vision settled down and (apart from a very transient attack of blurred vision lasting a couple of days shortly afterwards) no further disturbance of vision has been reported at all.

Case 31   Female, aged 17   Inexplicable permanent refractive change

The prescription found when this young lady was first tested was:

> R 6/36 – 1.75/ – 0.25 × 50 6/5
> L 6/60 – 3.75DS 6/5

She came for regular refractive checks during the next two or three years, during which time there was no significant change. She now came in complaining of recent headaches, and the prescription for the left eye had altered to:

   L – 1.75DS 6/5

The R refraction was practically unaltered, and again no signs of any pathology was discovered. She was referred, and the surgeon she saw was very puzzled by the change. He said that the diagnosis was extremely doubtful, but that he had decided to treat it on the basis of a suspected optic neuritis. The patient had already been attending her GP, incidentally, but her only problem, so far as she knew, was overweight. Six months later she came in again for refraction, when no change in the power or acuity was found. Her general health remained good.

However, the myopia continued to reduce, and three years later the prescription had altered to:

   R 6/60 – 2.00/ – 0.25 × 60 6/5
   L 6/9 – 0.75/ – 0.25 × 10 6/5

Her general health was still good, and no explanation has been found to account for the vast change in refraction in her left eye. Such cases are rare, but all practitioners encounter them from time to time. In the majority of cases, of course, there is a pathological underlying cause, and one must always be on the look-out for this possibility.

Case 32   Male, aged 52   Refractive change due to Meibomian cyst

An occasional reason for an apparently inexplicable unilateral refractive change – and one which can very easily be overlooked – is a meibomian cyst in the upper lid. In this respect the following case is instructive:

   R 6/9 +   + 1.00/ – 0.50 × 170 6/5
   L 6/9 +   + 1.00/ – 0.50 × 175 6/5   Add + 1.50 reading

Just under a year after having this prescription dispensed the patient returned, complaining of blurring with his right eye. There was no pain or discomfort. A small cyst could be felt in the R upper lid. These often occur without disturbing the refraction, but in this case there was a definite change. The R refraction had now altered to:

   R 6/12 + 0.75/ – 1.00 × 130 6/9 (variable)

After a prolonged course of warm saline bathing the cyst finally resolved, and the refraction and acuity returned almost exactly to their original levels.

If large or bizarre refractive changes are found in a patient – especially if he has not been examined in your practice before – it can be due to any one of a number of causes. The simplest explanation, which should be checked out before anything else, is that they have not produced their most recent pair of spectacles. Or perhaps these have been wrongly focimetered by your assistant? But if there is any doubt about the change, be very careful. Look for signs of underlying disorder, and refer if there is any doubt. Even if everything seems in order, it may be a good idea to ask the patient to return in a week or so's time for rechecking before undertaking any dispensing.

19.3   Errors in writing down, prescribing, or dispensing

It is very important to write all prescription details neatly and clearly, both on the record and on order forms, in order to minimize errors. Even so, mistakes do sometimes occur, and lenses must always be checked meticulously before handing out. If a patient returns with a complaint, the prescription should be checked against the details on the record card for the satisfaction of both parties.

It may be asked how some of the errors categorized in this series could possibly have got past the checking stage. I am unable to explain how or why they occurred, but can only say that they are real examples – they actually happened – and the details recorded here should be a warning against over-confidence. We all make mistakes, but should endeavour to ensure that they are put right at the earliest possible stage.

Case 33   Female, aged 57

This patient had been examined elsewhere only just over a month before. She had been prescribed R and L – 0.25DS in a pale tint for reading, but had found them to be completely useless. She returned to the prescriber, but was told she must get used to them, and no attempt was made to investigate the reason for her complaint at this stage. She complained to the FPC, who authorised a re-examination. The refraction was then found to be:

    R – 0.25DS 6/5
    L – 0.25 cyl H 6/5   Add + 1.75 reading

It was quite evident that she had been supplied with distance lenses instead of reading, but that the substance of her complaints had just not been listened to.

Case 34   Female, aged 78

This was another case where spectacles had been supplied with which the patient was unable to see. She had returned several times to complain, but had simply been told that she must 'persevere', and would eventually get used to them. It was not until her third or fourth visit that somebody took the trouble to focimeter the lenses supplied, when she was told 'Sorry, one of our staff inadvertently ordered them plus instead of minus'. The lenses were then changed, when she found them at least wearable, but she was still not comfortable with the prescription, and had understandably lost confidence in the expertise of the organization concerned. She therefore now came for a second opinion. She was wearing the prescription as just replaced:

R $- 1.00/ - 2.50 \times 15$
L $- 2.50/ - 3.00 \times 175$ Add $+ 3.50$ reading

It would have been nice to think that after such a disastrous mistake, special care would have been taken to ensure that the best vision possible had been obtained with the corrected prescription. But re-examination now showed that the cylinder axes had been carelessly set:

R $- 1.00/ - 1.75 \times 25$ $6/9 +$
L $- 2.00/ - 2.00 \times 150$ $6/9 +$ Add $+ 3.25$ reading

Case 35   Male, aged 30

This was a patient who had moved to this district from his home town many miles away. He was aware that he had a complicated prescription, so he wrote to his previous prescriber for details. He received the following 'copy' of the glasses originally supplied:

R $+ 2.00/ - 0.25 \times H$
L $+ 0.50/ - 0.50 \times 10$

These were duly made up locally, but he found them uncomfortable and quite impossible to get on with. He returned several times to the practice where he had obtained them to complain, but was simply told that they were 'correct in accordance with the prescription' – which they were. He tried to explain that he knew that they must be wrong, because 'the right lens in my old prescription was much thicker at the top and the bottom'. Incredibly, this failed to produce any reaction from the supplier, and the patient of course sought advice elsewhere. The prescription was found to be:

R $+ 2.25/ - 6.00 \times 10$ 2^Δ Up $6/9$
L $+ 1.00/ - 0.75 \times H$ $6/5$

What must have happened was that the prescription sent to him had been carelessly copied, and 0.25 cyl written down instead of 6.25 cyl.

Case 36   Female, aged 65

This was a case of a high, but relatively simple prescription which the patient found exceedingly uncomfortable to wear. The powers were R and L – 13.00DS, but had been dispensed with the centres 5mm too wide apart. The higher the power, of course, the more important it is to have the centres correctly set. In this instance the effective decentration was producing unwanted base-in prism of about 6.5 prism dioptres and it was rather surprising that her complaint was of discomfort but not of diplopia.

Case 37   Female, aged 39

This was a similar instance, involving lower power but larger decentration. The patient had had her spectacles 'copied' while on holiday abroad, and was delighted to get them extraordinarily cheaply. 'But the trouble is, though I can see perfectly clearly with them, everything keeps going double'.

Her prescription was approximately R and L + 4.00DS, and they had been dispensed with a DCD of 70 instead of 60. In this case, of course, the induced prism was base-out, and increased when close work was attempted because of the narrower interpupillary distance.

Case 38   Female, aged 17

This young lady had been refracted in another area only two months previously. Her prescription was altered, but she was experiencing persistent ocular discomfort and aching pains over her eyes. The prescription supplied was checked and found to be quite correct:

$$R - 2.00/ - 1.00 \times V \ 6/4$$
$$L - 1.25/ - 0.25 \times 105 \ 6/4$$
$$1^{\Delta} \ \text{Exo distance.} \ 2^{\Delta} \ \text{Exo near}$$

Unfortunately for her, these lenses had been dispensed in a huge frame, and the DCD was 75 mm. As her PD was only 62 mm, she had the equivalent of approximately 3^{Δ} base-in incorporated in her prescription. Immediately after the lenses were replaced, correctly centred, her symptoms disappeared completely.

Incidentally, it should be realized that the patient who is esophoric only diverges his eyes to the primary position, when taking up binocular vision. If an individual is made 'artificially esophoric' by the introduction of base-in prism, he has to go beyond this point into a true divergence, which is much more likely to induce discomfort.

Case 39   Male, aged 51

This case serves to emphasize the point made above. Spectacles recently supplied had proved to be unwearable, although they were very similar in power to the pair he already had. The prescription was:

R -1.50DS 6/5
L $-1.00/-0.25 \times$ H 6/5

His actual PD was 60 mm, and the original lenses were centred to 61 mm. But the latest pair had a DCD of 75 mm, because the frame supplied was too large and no consideration had been given to centration. He had about 6Δ of esophoria at distance, which he could normally overcome, but the additional induced base-in prism due to the DCD was too much for comfort. This was verified by placing 2^Δ base-out in front of his later spectacles, which he immediately said provided relief.

Case 40   Male, aged 54

This man had been refracted only nine months before, and supplied with bifocals. One of his complaints was that he had ordered tinted lenses, but they had been supplied in clear glass, but this was the least of his optical problems. The prescription supplied, near enough correct, was:

R $-5.75/-1.25 \times 165$ 6/5 +
L $-3.25/-0.50 \times 160$ 6/5 +   Add $+2.00$ reading
$\frac{1}{2}^\Delta$ L Hyperphoria 2^Δ Exophoria dist

In anisometropic prescriptions such as this, the vertical centrations are as important as the horizontal, and if separate pairs are supplied, they should more or less coincide with the pupil centres. But this patient required bifocals for his work, and they had been made up as ordinary 22 mm round segment solids, with the centres level and above datum. His distance PD was 64 mm, but the distance DCD given was 72 mm. Even this might have been tolerated had the segments been well inset, but the inset was in fact only 1 mm in each eye!

He had not returned to the prescriber to complain, but had simply reverted to his previous pair of spectacles, which were not at all strong enough for close work. He was told that he should have gone back much earlier, and demanded a replacement. His reply was illuminating. He was a technical man himself, he said, and he considered it too much to expect that an individual who had produced such unsatisfactory work could be trusted to put it right. Yet the refraction had been careful and accurate; in this case it was good work sabotaged by careless dispensing.

Segment setting

Errors in segment setting are unfortunately not uncommon. Segment height is a difficult area because no setting is ideal for all purposes, and patients' complaints often revolve round a particular task for which bifocals are unsuited. Some practitioners tend to err on the low side, because too high a setting is intolerable. However, many patients adapt easily if the setting is a *little* high, by slightly altering their head position. If they are set appreciably low, on the other hand, reading becomes uncomfortable because the head has to be tilted back into an unnatural position.

One would not expect much discrepancy in insetting, as this is directly related to the patient's PD and habitual working distance. Nevertheless, instances are often seen of incorrect horizontal setting – almost invariably too wide, because too large a frame has been chosen. Occasionally one sees bifocals with no inset, and I have even seen a pair (which were being worn with very little pleasure) in which the segments had been decentred out instead of in! In another instance (which was however picked up at the checking stage) the dispenser noticed that the engraved location markings were on the same side of each lens; both had been selected from varifocal blanks intended for the left eye. The lenses had arrived marked up with the checking circles in their theoretically correct positions, but on one of them the marking did not coincide with the reading centre at all; in effect one lens had been decentred in for reading and the other decentred out.

Ensuring that the maximum plus has been obtained

Binocular additions

When performing refractions it is wise to bear in mind the patient's symptoms and reason for seeking advice. The next two examples, involving eyestrain after close work but initially almost no refractive error, are instructive.

Case 41   Female, aged 17

This young lady was employed on sewing and upholstery work, and complained of frequent headaches and eyestrain. The refraction initially indicated low myopia:

> R 6/9 + (– 0.50)/ – 0.25 × 140 6/6 +
> L 6/9 + (– 0.25)/ – 0.25 × 10 6/6 +
> $2\frac{1}{2}^{\Delta}$ Exophoria distance 5^{Δ} Exophoria near

The refraction and acuity tended to fluctuate, giving rise to a suspicion of ciliary cramp or pseudo-myopia. It was noticed that she held the reading chart at an excessively close distance. She was therefore rechecked binocularly, with particular efforts made to see if she would accept binocular additions. It was necessary to spend some time on this, but eventually she accepted a full + 0.75DS binocular addition (it is rare to find more than 0.50DS), with which she could still read 6/6 + . Now that some relaxation of accommodation had occurred, the near exophoria was checked again, when it was found to have increased to $8^\triangle$. It was decided to order the fullest correction found, and to incorporate weak base-in prisms in the prescription. She was also told that it was very important for her to work further out.

Had the prescription originally indicated by the preliminary refraction been dispensed, her symptoms would have been aggravated instead of relieved.

Case 42   Female, aged 14

This was a similar case involving eyestrain with close work, and again there was a habit of reading at too close a distance. Initial refraction was:

R 6/5 + 0.25/ – 0.25 × V 6/5
L 6/6 + + 0.25/ – 0.50 × V 6/5
$2\frac{1}{2}^\triangle$ Esophoria distance $6^\triangle$ Esophoria near

It was evident that if this represented the whole of her refractive error, spectacles were unlikely to make the slightest impact on her visual symptoms. Binocular additions were tried, but not at first accepted. Attempts were then made to relax accommodation, by giving her print to read through plus additions; these were removed after a few moments and she was returned to the distance chart. The next method tried was to direct her to the distance chart, and to put in base-out prisms of moderate power ($4^\triangle$, increasing to $6^\triangle$ when it had been established that she could maintain binocular vision). She was encouraged to try to see the letters clearly, after which a weak binocular addition was inserted, and the prisms then removed. The principle involved was to try to build up convergence in excess of accommodation, and then to see if when convergence was relaxed an associated relaxation of accommodation would occur. (Effectively, it was exercising positive relative convergence.)

After some minutes she was able to maintain clear vision for short periods with a + 0.50DS binocular addition. This confirmed the existence of ciliary cramp and justified prescribing the full prescription found for close work. Cases requiring build-up of plus like this are usually encountered in young people, but even in older age groups a small increase in one or both the eyes is sometimes found if efforts are made to reveal it.

Case 43   Female, aged 72

Vague symptoms of visual discomfort had been experienced by this patient for a considerable time. She had been examined fairly recently but had been told that there was insufficient change to warrant altering her spectacles. The old pair were:

R + 2.25/ – 0.25 × 75
L + 2.50/ – 0.50 × 55   Add + 2.50 reading

On re-examination the initial prescription found was:

R + 2.25/ – 0.50 × 105 6/6 +
L + 2.75/ – 0.50 × 85 6/5   Add + 2.50 reading

With these lenses there was exactly 0.25 red dominance on monocular bichromatic tests with either eye, and there also seemed to be good binocular balance. To ensure that the accommodation had been fully relaxed, and that the tests had been clearly understood, the bichromatic tests were repeated, but with the occluder removed and replaced by a + 1.75DS alternately before each eye. With the left eye no difference was found, but the R then accepted a full additional + 0.25DS to obtain the same degree of red dominance. This result was supported by the fact that near binocular balance was obtained with equal reading additions.

For elderly persons who spend much of their time indoors, the effects of a convex prescription which is 0.25 weak, or a concave prescription which is 0.25 too strong, are exaggerated, because for most of the day they do not fully relax accommodation in distance viewing. Another factor influencing comfort here was the change in cylinder axis; had this been the only change it would not have been significant, but there was also a difference in power.

One other point could be mentioned here; if unequal reading additions are found although the distance acuities are practically equal, *always* check back to ensure that the distance refraction is still in balance.

Case 44   Male, aged 69

One frequently encounters cases where the precise spherical or cylindrical component should really be a one-eighth power, and a decision has to be made whether to round up or down to the nearest 0.25. In the present instance, the preliminary result was:

R 6/6 – – 0.75/ – 0.25 × 135 6/6 +
L 6/9 + – 0.25/ – 0.50 × 65 6/5   Add R + 2.50; L + 2.25 reading
Ocular muscle balance normal

With the above correction in place he gave red dominance of exactly 0.37 with the right eye and 0.25 with the left on monocular bichromatic tests. This suggested that the true spherical element with the right eye should be 0.62 instead of 0.75.

However, when binocular balancing was checked using polarized targets it was necessary to reduce the initial basic prescription for the right eye by 0.25.

This was confusing, because it indicated that the R sphere should be – 0.50. When this small reduction was made, near binocular balance was achieved with equal reading additions. It was therefore decided to make the R sphere 0.50 and to give equal reading additions of + 2.25DS. If doubt remains in cases like this it is useful to apply rapid alternate occlusion with an extra + 0.25DS first before one eye and then before the other. If preference is consistently expressed for the vision in the eye without the extra + 0.25 addition then it can be assumed that the prescription will be comfortable.

Minor fluctuations in refraction can occur at any time, and one cannot always expect to find reasons for apparent discrepancies in test results. In the case above, however, it will be noted that the R acuity was not quite so good as the left, and this may have induced slight accommodative efforts in an attempt to obtain better vision. (*Note*: I have emphasized the need to elicit the fullest plus (or minimal minus) in refracting patients, but this must not be adopted so rigidly that over-corrections are given. Each practitioner comes to develop his own particular method for finalizing his prescription, but if proper care is taken the end results are virtually identical. My own technique is to endeavour to finish up with + 0.12 or + 0.25 red dominance on the distance bichromatic tests, and then to reduce the prescription by 0.25 overall (in the case of minus prescriptions, of course, to *increase* it by 0.25 overall). This eliminates the slight over-correction which otherwise would result from tests carried out at six metres.)

Prescribing for reading

Reading spectacles are usually associated with presbyopia, but it must be remembered that many young hypermetropes wear their theoretical distance correction almost exclusively for reading, and this has to be borne in mind when deciding what to prescribe. Younger adults often prefer a slight reduction of convex power (except where very low prescriptions are concerned) because a full strength pair of glasses, only worn occasionally, may cause blurring or discomfort at distance. The older pre-presbyope, on the other hand, will usually benefit from the full prescription, because he is verging on the need for a reading addition.

Case 45   Female, aged 30

This patient had worn glasses regularly, but only for close work, since she was at school. The refraction was:

R + 1.75/ – 0.50 × 160 6/5
L + 1.75/ – 0.50 × 150 6/5

Retinoscopy had confirmed that there was at least this amount of hypermetropia, but some ciliary cramp was present, and the prescription had to be built up by binocular refraction. She moved to another area and had new spectacles prescribed:

$$R \ +1.00/-0.50 \times 175$$
$$L \ +1.00/-0.50 \times 150$$

With these she complained of persistent asthenopia and headaches. Re-examination showed that the original prescription was still in fact correct, though there was still some difficulty in uncovering the maximum plus as mentioned before. The probability was that she had been refracted too quickly, not allowing enough time for accommodation to relax.

Case 46   Female, aged 29

This case was brought before an Ophthalmic Investigation Committee following a complaint by the patient alleging unneccessary prescribing. The prescription issued was:

$$R \ 6/6 \ +0.25/+0.25 \times 95 \ 6/6$$
$$L \ 6/6 - \ +0.50DS \ 6/6$$

It was stated that she found these lenses blurred her vision at distance, and after several return visits she consulted another practitioner, who said that he did not consider she needed spectacles. It was not very clear why she had sought an eye examination in the first place, though she did mention that her eyes were sensitive to light, and the prescription had been made up in a pale tint.

The practitioner originally consulted was cleared of any breach of his terms of service, but the case highlights one of the difficult areas in prescribing, and the need for circumspection in correcting very low refractive errors. Asked to justify the issuing of this prescription, he said that he had told the patient that there was only a small refractive error, and that spectacles would not improve the acuity, though they might relieve her discomfort in bright light. She was employed on clerical work, and many practitioners might well have thought she would perhaps derive some benefit from the weak plus correction.

There is no doubt that some patients would have found close work more comfortable with it, especially if they were about ten years older. Prescribing anything weaker than this (R and L +0.25DS, for example) can be defended only with considerable difficulty, but such instances do occasionally arise, as the next example shows.

Case 47   Female, aged 26

This illustrates how dependent a patient can become if in a nervous state and worried about her eyes. This lady was in poor health and constantly apprehensive because her fiancé was in a hazardous occupation. She had seen another OO, 18 months before, who had prescribed two pairs:

$$R \quad +0.25/-0.50 \times H$$
$$L \quad +0.25/-0.25 \times H$$

Add $+0.50$ reading

She wore the weaker pair regularly and put on the reading pair whenever close work was involved. She had marked photophobia and some weakness of convergence, but accommodation was only slightly depressed when I saw her. I considered it most unsatisfactory to supply a reading pair with such a weak addition in the circumstances. Instead, she was provided with one pair of spectacles for general wear – very similar in power to the 'distance' pair she was already wearing – but incorporating weak base-in prisms to assist convergence. She was also referred to her GP for a check on her general health.

When next seen, seven years later, she was still in poor health, but was at least still managing with one pair of spectacles. She had been supplied with R and L $+0.25 \times 90$, in a pale tint, without any prismatic element. She insisted that they were a great help to her, and that she could not possibly manage without them. Unfortunately, this was true, though her dependence was really psychological and not visual; it would have been useless to contradict in the circumstances.

Very rarely, one finds cases where dependence on a low prescription is associated with weakened accommodation, and it is advisable to check this.

Prescribing for presbyopia

After the distance prescription has been ascertained, consideration has to be given to the reading addition required. There are many ways or dealing with this apparently simple problem, not all of which are entirely satisfactory. There is a tendency to rely heavily on near bichromatic tests nowadays, yet it is surprising how accurate a balance can be achieved simply by using a reading chart with very small print (N.4.5 for preference) and alternate cover. The amount of addition depends mainly on the amplitude of accommodation and the patient's habitual working distance, but there are a number of other factors to be considered, some of which will be discussed in the cases which follow.

The young optometrist of today has no conception of the arguments that raged around the interpretation of near bichromatic tests in the mid 1950s or thereabouts. Should equality of red and green be taken as the criterion, or did this tend to produce over-correction? What is the 'average' reading distance? And do you estimate the near addition from the middle of the patient's average range, or at some closer distance?

These points are not without relevance today. Getting the addition just right – or as near as practically possible – is a very important matter indeed. How important is soon brought home to a prescriber who has to replace an expensive pair of bifocals because he has over or underestimated the reading power required!

Influence of previous precription

Case 48   Female, aged 48

In the course of case history taking, this patient stated that she had never been tested or had glasses before. The prescription was quite simple and straightforward:

> R 6/6 +1.00DS 6/5
> L 6/6 +1.00/−0.25 × 45 6/5   Add +1.00 reading

This reading addition erred a little on the weak side, which I considered advisable as she had not worn glasses before. But when I came to refract her husband, immediately afterwards, I found that he was wearing R and L +1.75DS, which would obviously have also suited her very well. On questioning her it transpired that she did in fact borrow them regularly for reading, and she added that they had not seemed quite so good lately. The reading addition for her new spectacles was therefore increased to +1.25 to take this into account.

The fact that 'I've not been tested before', does not necessarily mean 'I've not worn glasses before' is of especial importance now that 'ready-made reading glasses' have once again become available to the public. Patients who select the reading prescription they think suits them from a display in a store almost invariably choose lenses which are too strong having regard to their accommodation. So that when, later on, they visit an optometrist who prescribes, however carefully, for a reasonable reading range while still ensuring they have some accommodation in play, they return to complain that they 'get more magnification' with their old, cheap pair. Much tact and patience is needed because, though they will often admit that the range is wrong, it is difficult to convince them that extending the range invariably reduces the magnification.

Case 49   Female, aged 59

This was another instance in which misleading information was given by the patient. She produced her old pair of spectacles, and complained that she had not been able to get a satisfactory pair for some years. Focimeter readings were:

R + 2.00/ – 0.25 × 90
L + 2.00/ – 0.25 × 80

After examination the refraction was found to be:

R + 0.50/ – 0.25 × 85 6/5
L + 0.50/ – 0.25 × 65 6/5   Add + 2.00 reading

Ocular muscle balance was normal and convergence good. As her old pair seemed so weak, although she had previously been tested quite recently, she was questioned more closely. It then transpired that the pair she had brought in had been supplied a very long time ago, but she preferred them because 'they don't blur so much at distance as the latest pair.'

It was disconcerting to discover that the genuine 'latest pair' was of almost exactly the same prescription as that just found. Evidently the slight increase in distance blur with the extra + 0.50 addition was more than she could tolerate. Some time was spent explaining the problem to her, and it was decided to supply the full prescription in half-eye spectacles, which proved to be entirely satisfactory.

Incidentally, it is always advisable to explain to presbyopic patients that they will get blurring at distance through their reading glasses. This may seem so obvious to the practitioner that he may not bother to mention it, but if the patient is forewarned a potential source of trouble is immediately eliminated.

Case 50   Female, aged 75

In this example, the fact that the old spectacles brought in were incorrect was not the fault of the patient. Their prescription was:

R + 3.25DS
L + 3.75DS

She just happened to mention, in conversation, that she had also been supplied with a duplicate pair, which had always seemed more comfortable and clearer. Hints like this should not be ignored, and she was asked to produce this spare pair for comparison, when although the dioptric powers were found to be identical, $1\frac{1}{2}^\Delta$ base in had been incorporated into each lens, so it was certainly not a true duplicate. The refraction now was:

R + 0.50/ – 0.50 × 90 6/9
L + 0.75/ – 0.25 × 40 6/9 +   Add + 3.00 reading (minimum)
4^Δ Exophoria distance 14^Δ Exophoria near

This high near exophoria was accompanied by weak convergence, so it was decided to incorporate 3^Δ base in into each lens of the reading glasses. Ideally, she would have benefited from a higher reading addition, but this would have entailed an appreciable increase in the amount of base-in prism required. Weight and appearance must always be balanced against minor improvements in magnification, particularly in view of the current preference for large eye sizes.

Low myopia and presbyopia

Myopes of low degree often read without their spectacles, especially as presbyopia approaches. If their distance error increases, it can produce problems, as illustrated in the next example:

Case 51   Female, aged 60

This patient was wearing R – 1.50DS L – 0.75DS. She had been prescribed spectacles more recently to the following prescription:

> R – 2.00DS
> L – 1.25DS

She was not at all happy with these because, she said, 'They made reading worse'. Yet this later pair were in fact approximately correct, as the refraction now was:

> R – 2.00/ – 0.25 × 80 6/5
> L – 1.00/ – 0.25 × 90 6/5   Add + 2.25 reading

When she had been less myopic and only slightly presbyopic there was no problem because she could get by with the weaker distance pair for general purposes, and even if she left them off the left distance vision would have been passable. Occasionally an increase in myopia at this age results from efforts to continue to read without glasses as presbyopia increases, putting considerable strain on the accommodation, because when the visual problems are resolved the myopia sometimes decreases later on. In the case under discussion it was explained to the patient that the only real solution would be to have bifocals, and these proved to be quite satisfactory in practice.

Case 52   Male, aged 50

This was a similar case to the above. Until his present visit, he had only worn distance spectacles, and had been taking them off to read for a considerable time. He realized that this was unsatisfactory, and requested bifocals at the commencement of the consultation. Refraction was quite straightforward:

> R – 2.25/ – 0.50 × 95 6/6 +
> L – 2.50/ – 0.50 × 85 6/6 +   (Add + 1.00DS reading)

When assessing the reading prescription it is important to emphasize to the patient that you need to know the distance at which he *prefers* to work – not simply the clearest position at which he can see print with the prescription inserted in the trial frame. A complication arose because he was very definite that he wished to read at about 40 cm, for which the + 1.00DS addition would have been correct. But as he had been reading without glasses for two or three *years* (effectively giving himself a + 2.25DS reading addition) it was thought unwise to make it so low. It was explained that he would have difficulty inside this range, and might find he still had to take off the glasses for any fine work. The reading addition was accordingly increased to + 1.50DS, a modification which was well justified as he adapted to the bifocals without any difficulty.

When prescribing for low myopic presbyopes, it is essential to consider just what the effect of the prescription will be in any individual case. Next we have an instance in which bifocals were definitely not a good idea.

Case 53   Female, aged 56

This lady had been refracted some years before, and was wearing bifocals to the following prescription:

$$R \; -1.25/-0.50 \times 180$$
$$L \; -1.00/-0.50 \times 180$$
Add + 0.75 reading

These, she insisted, had never been satisfactory. 'I could always see better for reading if I took them off'. She had been in the habit of reading without glasses anyway, and a moment's thought will show that the prescriber was indeed making her near vision worse with this very low reading addition. With the passage of time, she had become more presbyopic, as the refraction now indicated:

$$R \; 6/24 \quad -1.50/-0.75 \times 180 \; 6/6 +$$
$$L \; 6/36 \quad -1.50/-0.50 \times 5 \; 6/6$$
Add + 1.75 reading

Even now, of course, the reading addition only more or less neutralized the distance prescription, and would not have made any real improvement in her reading vision. It was therefore suggested that she should have only a distance pair at this stage, with which she was quite satisfied. Had she insisted on bifocals, it would probably have been wise to increase the reading addition to + 2.00DS, so that at least she could not again say that close work was actually worse with the spectacles supplied.

Insufficient reading addition

The need for accuracy in prescribing and dispensing bifocals should not need to be stressed, but it does. Inaccurate segment setting is the most common problem, and would occur much less often if the fitting was always checked carefully when spectacles were collected.

Case 54   Male, aged 73

This man had been seen regularly at a practice in another area, but on the latest occasion he had been most dissatisfied with the bifocals supplied and had returned with them several times. He complained in particular that his reading range was too long, and that the vision of his left eye seemed worse than that of the right. He was annoyed that no attempt was made to recheck his vision, though the optician concerned did change the frame. This did not make any improvement, and he had got into the habit of taking his glasses off to read, which he had never done in the past.

When his spectacles were focimetered the main reason for his difficulty was obvious:

$$R - 5.75/ - 0.50 \times 80 \ 6/6 +$$
$$L - 6.25/ - 1.00 \times 90 \ 6/6 \ partly \qquad Add \ + 1.00 \ reading$$

The distance refraction was correct, but of course he could not read at his age with an addition of only + 1.00DS. Evidently the practitioner to whom he had returned had assumed that whatever problems there were must be due simply to the segment setting – presumably that was why he had changed the frame. Undoubtedly the weak addition was due to an error in ordering or manufacture, because an individual who could get the distance prescription right in a refractive error of this type was obviously capable of assessing the addition correctly. This leads up to a cardinal rule in dealing with complaints: *never assume that the prescription on the record card in your hand is the same as the one in the spectacles the patient is wearing.*

Anisometropia and incipient presbyopia

From time to time one encounters patients who have learned to use unorthodox methods in order to come to terms with their visual dificulties, and they tend to present special problems to the prescriber when they come for advice.

Case 55   Male, aged 45

This patient was wearing:

R – 6.25DS
L – 5.25DS

The actual refractive error was:

R – 7.50DS 6/6 +
L – 5.00DS 6/6 +

He was a medical practitioner and fully understood the nature of his visual problems. He was a little presbyopic and was obviously using the right eye for reading and the left for distance. He insisted that he was perfectly satisfied with this expedient and did not want bifocals. It is a mistake to try to alter a person's habits if they are content with them; the amount of blur on the R side was not excessive, and in any case the R accommodation was somewhat weaker than the L – probably because it had been undercorrected for a long time.

As he grew older, however, the right eye became much more myopic, creating new difficulties. By the age of 60, the refraction had altered to:

R – 10.00/ – 0.75 95 6/6
L – 5.75/ – 0.50 85 6/6 +   Add + 2.50DS reading

He was not at all happy now if the right eye was reduced sufficiently to give clear reading vision, because he still retained binocular vision and this degree of unilateral blur bothered him. Separate pairs were tried, but after a few months he discarded the reading pair and read without – now of course using his other eye for close work.

Unequal reading additions

Small differences in R and L reading additions often require to be made, but one must not make a drastic increase on one side simply because that eye has poorer vision, as this would result in unequal working distances. There are occasionally special instances, however, where this can be of benefit to the patient.

Case 56 Female, aged 48

This patient had had bilateral operations for glaucoma, and there was an old-standing oblique strabismus of about 7 degrees, but visual acuity was excellent:

R 6/60 – 2.00DS 6/5
L 6/9 + + 0.50/ – 0.50 × 55 6/5   Add R + 1.50 L + 1.75 for reading

The L accommodation was about 1.00D weaker than the R. She did not have binocular vision and used her R eye for distance and the L for reading.

Bifocals are definitely unsuitable for this type of case, so separate distance and reading spectacles were dispensed. It may be wondered why, if the accommodation in the left eye was full 1.00DS weak, only 0.25 difference was made between the reading additions. The reason for this was that as she normally used her right eye almost exclusively for reading the *relatively* weak addition prescribed for the left eye would give her the advantage of better intermediate vision when this was required.

It would not have been practicable to supply one pair of spectacles with a distance lens in one eye and a reading lens in the other – after all, this was the situation she had if she did not wear glasses at all, and she certainly did not find this satisfactory. Hers was an 'essentially alternating' type of squint, in which the two eyes work entirely independently. When wearing her distance correction, she could obtain good vision on either side by 'alternating' if the need arose – an expedient to which she would frequently resort to while driving, for instance.

19.4   Where visual acuity does not improve as expected

The preliminary examination usually provides a rough indication of the visual acuity that will be obtained. With an adult patient who enjoys good health and binocular vision, one would anticipate R and L 6/5 with correction if the fundi and media appear normal. If vision does not improve as anticipated, especial care must be taken to check for errors in prescribing or possible pathological factors. Before embarking on any complex investigations, however, the simplest and most obvious sources of trouble should be eliminated; thumb marks on the trial lenses, smears on the mirror if an indirect chart is used, or the lenses set so close to the eyes that they touch the lashes, for instance.

(Sometimes the refraction shows no change, and the acuity is normal, but the patient insists that his vision is not clear with the spectacles supplied. Invariably the prescription must be checked; apart from possible dispensing errors there have been instances of the wrong pair having been handed out. Complaints of blurred vision can also arise because of scratching of the lenses, or the peculiar hazing that results from careless use of hair lacquer spray – the latter often needing special solvents for its removal.)

The examples which follow cannot cover all eventualities, but are a representative selection of real case histories which illustrate some of the wide variety of problems which may be encountered.

Case 57   Male, aged 65   Floating opacities

The complaint here was of occasional blurring of vision. He was wearing:

R – 2.00DS
L – 2.25DS   Add + 2.00 reading

(Ocular muscle balance normal, both for distance and near vision)
The refraction showed only a small increase:

R – 2.50/ – 0.25 × 65 6/9 + (variable)   Add R + 2.50DS
L – 2.25/ – 0.50 × 85 6/6 +   L + 2.25DS

The R acuity varied intermittently during the sight test. It was never worse than 6/9 but he could not quite achieve 6/6 at best. He was asked to look in different directions and then forward again, which maximized the fluctuations in acuity. He had some fine vitreous opacities which, although they had seemed negligible during ophthalmoscopy, tended to float across his line of vision and proved to be the cause of the transient blurring which had bothered him. It will be noted that with both the old and new prescriptions he did not really require any assistance for reading, but he preferred bifocals for his work. It was considered quite justifiable to dispense new lenses, because the disturbance from floating opacities is generally minimized when the sharpest visual acuity is achieved; also the amount of increase with the right eye – equal to – 0.50/ – 0.25 – was sufficient of itself to make replacement worthwhile.

Unilateral lowering of acuity due to microtropia

Case 58   Female, aged 21

This patient had been examined by another practitioner only seven months previously, and was worried about her eyes. She had returned several times, complaining of lachrymation and irritation, together with the fact that she had noticed that one eye did not see quite so well as the other. Refraction gave:

R 6/24 + 0.50/ – 1.50 × 170 1^Δ base in 6/12 +
L 6/9 +   – 0.50 × 20 6/6 +
1^Δ Esophoria. Ortho V dist. 2^Δ Esophoria near vision C.N.P. 17–19 cm

She was wearing practically the same prescription as the above except that the prism prescribed for the right eye was $\frac{1}{2}^\Delta$ base up. To investigate the poor acuity the cover test was applied, but no movement could be detected objectively. She was therefore invited to look at the distance spotlight with both eyes open, and the right eye was suddenly covered, when she was asked if she could detect any movement, however slight. As expected, she did not (because she was fixing with her good eye), but when the test was repeated, and the left eye covered, she reported a small but definite upward shift of the spotlight. She obtained normal binocular vision and stereoscopy, although this minute deviation demonstrated that the right eye was not fixing truly centrally when both eyes were in use; in other words, she had a R microtropia. There was no point in attempting to correct this – it was her normal habit of vision and was not associated with any vertical phoria. Having regard to the receded convergence near point, it was more important to give some relief to this, which was why the base-in prism was prescribed.

What was needed in this case, as in so many other examples of complaints which arise, was an explanation. There can be little doubt but that the R acuity must have been poorer than the L from her earliest years, but it had not bothered her until discomfort from her spectacles, and perhaps other sources of irritation as well, had made her more introspective and worried about her sight. At all events, her symptoms disappeared after her spectacles were changed and the reason for the differences in acuities had been made clear to her.

Minute macular lesion

Case 59   Male, aged 64

On previous visits the acuities had been been excellent at R and L 6/5. He had become worried about some deterioration in the vision of his left eye during the preceding fortnight, and said that there seemed to be a very small, faint bluish-grey shadow in his field of vision. One would naturally look for a macular lesion, but no signs were visible at this stage, even with the convergent light beam. The prescription is immaterial here; the refraction was virtually unchanged but the corrected vision was now R 6/6 + L 6/18, with slight distortion of the letters seen with the left eye; he said that the outer letters in the 6/24 line were more distinct than the centre one. A very meticulous investigation of the central area with the Bjerrum screen revealed a minute paracentral scotoma, located at 35 degrees up and out, but so close to the fixation point that it was practically touching. It was absolute only for a 2 mm white target at 1 metre, and it can easily be calculated that this subtends an angle slightly smaller than that of a 6/9 letter.

It is very easy to miss such cases in their earliest stages; he was of course referred and when next seen, only a month later, the suspected macular lesion had become visible and the acuity had deteriorated further in the affected eye.

Minute lesions higher in the visual pathway

In the case above the causative lesion was ocular, and would usually have been discernible on the initial examination. Visual disturbances due to lesions at a higher level than the optic disc may not be accompanied by any tell-tale signs, though those beyond the chiasma will usually be reflected as bilateral in their effects.

Case 60   Male, aged 76

This was basically only a routine re-visit for replacement reading spectacles, but the patient mentioned recent vague disturbances of his vision, and said that he thought things did not seem quite so clear to him. There were no significant ophthalmoscopic signs, and a small distance refractive correction improved his vision from R 6/18 L 6/12 to R 6/9 L 6/6. It must never be assumed, by the way, that if the patient is old, complaints about difficulties with his vision can be ignored, because 'it is bound to be poor at that age'.

In this case careful scotometry was also performed, which revealed at least two minute paracentral scotomata, which were homonymous and congruous, because they were still present when both eyes were unoccluded. One was 0.50 cm in diameter and just adjacent to the L of the fixation point and the other, 1.50 cm in diameter, was situated about 1½ degrees from the fixation point. It may be asked why, if the scotomata were homonymous, the visual acuity was better in the left eye. There were probably other factors influencing his vision at this advanced age, of course, but in any case results do not always conform to the pattern expected.

When an explanation of his symptoms can be given to the patient, he will usually be more prepared to live with it, even if no effective treatment is possible, because he will feel that his complaints have been listened to and given proper consideration and investigation.

Some logical sequence of eliminating tests must be applied in order to arrive at the reason for defective acuity. Unfortunately, the patient is unaware of the multifarious possible causes and tends to ascribe it (sometimes very aggressively) to his spectacles, if they have been supplied recently. The optometrist must guard against being tempted to put so much effort into attempts to improve on the refractive correction that he fails to give sufficient weight to other factors.

Case 61   Male, aged 70

This patient had been seen not long before by two other optometrists, who were concerned because his acuity could not be improved beyond a bare 6/9, whereas only a few weeks earlier it had been R and L 6/6 + . No signs could be detected in the fundi and the media were clear. It seemed highly unlikely that much further progress would result from going through the whole processes of examination and refraction again, especially as all the subjective findings were known to have been thoroughly checked.

It was considered that a different approach might prove more rewarding, and he was asked if he had noticed any peculiarity or difficulty with his eyes at or around the time the blurring had commenced – anything, it was emphasized, no matter how trivial or unimportant it may have been at the time. 'Well, yes', he replied, 'For a few days it seemed as if there was 'something funny' up on my left side somewhere – I couldn't tell you quite what it was, and anyway I don't notice it now'. This vague description provided the essential clue with the absolute minimum of time and effort. A central field check was then performed, which revealed a homonymous scotoma of moderate size in the upper left quadrant, extending just into the corresponding corner of the fixation area and thereby reducing the acuity to the level found.

It will be evident that 'vague symptoms' often reflect some underlying pathological condition, even though they may be only minor or transient, and their investigation sometimes produces surprising results.

Case 62   Female, aged 25

This lady had not had a 'sight test' before, as she greatly disliked the idea of having to wear spectacles, but eventually her symptoms drove her to seek advice:

$$R \ 6/9 \ +3.00/-0.50 \times 180 \ 6/9+$$
$$L \ 6/9 \ +2.75/-0.75 \times 180 \ 6/9+$$

Some ciliary cramp was present, which was assumed to account for the slightly reduced monocular acuity, but ocular 'muscle balance' was normal and she could read 6/5 binocularly. On a subsequent visit a small increase in plus was required. Visual acuity was very similar, and the eyes appeared normal on examination, but she expressed some concern about her eyes. It was not possible to ascertain precisely what the trouble was – she could not describe any definite symptoms – but there was no doubt that she sensed something was wrong. She was encouraged to define the reasons for her worries; there was still no positive lead, but she mentioned, among other things, an uncle who had lost his sight from some unspecified cause at a relatively early age. Scotometry was performed as a precaution, which revealed a small caeco-central scotoma. She was fully investigated after referral, when she was found to have toxic amblyopia and hypertension. These symptoms, the consultant considered, were due to her very heavy smoking habits (50 cigarettes daily) during the past few years. One would not expect to find tobacco amblyopia in a young female – the significant sign was only discovered because the conversation in case history taking had given rise to the suspicion that there might have been some complicating factors.

Misleading symptoms

On the other hand, it happens occasionally that the details given by the patient during case history taking are so meticulously described that they become wearying to listen to, or confusing factors are brought up which obscure the true picture. This last point is nicely illustrated in the next case.

Case 63   Female, aged 43

This patient had worn glasses for a short time as a schoolgirl, but had not had her eyes re-examined until now. A month previously, she had a severe cold, and had felt something splash into her eye while she was decorating her kitchen. She later visited her GP because the vision of her left eye seemed rather blurred. He referred her to the local eye hospital, when the possibility of frontal sinus infection was casually mentioned; an antibiotic was prescribed and she was discharged.

The blurring persisted, however, and she saw her GP again, when he recommended a 'sight test'. No signs were seen in the fundi, but it was noticed that the L pupillary reflexes were sluggish compared to the right. No distance refractive error was present, but visual acuity was R 6/5, L 6/12. Field investigations showed appreciable contraction with the left eye, and monocular testing of her colour vision revealed that this also was defective on the left side only. These signs suggested an attack of retro-bulbar neuritis, which was confirmed after referral. The chance coincidence of her getting something in her eye more or less at the same time as the infection commenced had been misleading.

Where there is recent acquired impairment of visual acuity it is a wise precaution to check all the main ocular functions, as hasty conclusions often result in error. ('Post hoc ergo propter hoc' reasoning works well enough to satisfy pigeons, as Skinner's experiments on conditioning have demonstrated so well, but optometry demands a much higher level of insight from its practitioners!)

Incidentally, this unilateral loss of colour vision can be most striking without the patient being aware of it, until it is brought to his notice during the examination. The next case, which also had misleading features because the eye which became affected had always had mild amblyopia associated with anisometropia, exemplifies this.

Case 64   Female, aged 47

On her previous visit, two years before, the prescription had been as below:

     R + 5.00/ – 1.25 × 95 6/9 +
     L + 2.75/ – 0.75 × 70 6/5
No appreciable ocular muscle imbalance

She now noticed blurring with her right eye subsequent to an attack of optic neuritis, and the acuity could not be improved beyond about 6/15 on that side. No significant fundus signs were visible at this stage, but she was unable to read any of the Ishihara plates with her right eye. The left retained normal colour vision. It will be realized that if she had been just a little more amblyopic before the attack, or the acuity slightly less impaired after it had occurred, the impact on vision could easily have passed unnoticed, as she had not realized colour discrimination had been affected. When re-examined three years later it was so marked that she thought the red streak produced by the Maddox rod before the right eye was white!

19.5   Difficult and grief cases

It is often difficult to decide whether or not a patient will benefit from spectacles, especially where low prescriptions or small changes are concerned. (Other factors can complicate the issues, such as a patient's irrational desire to wear spectacles, and complaints about the old pair being unsatisfactory and needing replacement, although no change has been found, may merely reflect an attempt to justify getting a more modern pair – what a psychiatrist has called 'preference masquerading as necessity'.) As a general rule, if it is doubtful whether spectacles will help, don't prescribe them.

Case 65   Female, aged 10   Pseudo myopia

This child complained of blurring of the writing on the blackboard at school, associated with headaches. Retinoscopy suggested about 1.0D of myopia, but results were unreliable. Refraction was difficult in spite of the simple prescription:

> R 6/24 – 0.25DS
> L 6/24 – 0.25DS   6/7.5 binocularly

Visual acuity fluctuated but was appreciably better if binocular viewing was allowed. The findings were quite inconsistent – clearly this negligible concave correction should not have produced this difference in acuity. Some esophoria was present, but the measured amount did not correlate with the cover test. Normal binocular vision and stereoscopy were present. She was handed the reading test card, which she held at only 14 to 15 cm from her eyes, which confirmed the suspicion of pseudo-myopia. It transpired that she had been reading in the waiting room at this close distance immediately prior to the sight test.

After a short delay to give her accommodation a chance to relax, she was taken back to the test chart, when she read R and L 6/9 + without lenses – evidently the induced ciliary cramp was already beginning to wear off. Spectacles were not of course prescribed, but her parents were told to ensure that she performed her close work at a more sensible distance in the future. Had the ciliary cramp been more persistent, of course, it would have been advisable to perform refraction under cycloplegia.

Malingering and hysterical amblyopia

Bizarre or inconsistent results, especially with children and young females, are not infrequently encountered and can be worrying to the practitioner, who should be prepared to consider the possibility of hysterical amblyopia or malingering. If he does not check for indications of these conditions, he may waste a lot of time and energy on a relatively simple case.

Case 66   Female, aged 10

The complaint in this case was of just not being able to see clearly. An examination 12 months before had shown a negligible hypermetropia and full 6/6 vision. She now read only R and L 6/9 partly, and the acuity did not improve with lenses. Retinoscopy showed virtually no error, confirmed by bichromatic tests in which – 0.25DS just gave green dominance. There was no deviation on cover tests. She said the near test type was so blurred that she could only attempt some of the words in the N 8 lines with difficulty. A plus addition was tried, but she said it was no clearer. This was highly suspicious; if she would read 6/9 at distance she should have been able to read small print with ease.

   Her visual acuity was rechecked, using a spare distance chart at varying distances, which confused her and produced acuity levels inconsistent with what should have been expected.

   She was sent out of the room and the situation was explained to her mother, who had been amazed at the child's apparent struggle to see. It transpired that she was at the top of her class at school, but recently her brother had been found to have defective vision in one eye, and had received much attention and sympathy on having to wear glasses. 'There's no doubt', her mother concluded, 'That she very much wants a pair of glasses and is prepared to try anything to get them'.

   The distinction between malingering and hysteria is often not sharp; the basic difference can be summed up briefly by saying that the hysteric deceives himself, and under test conditions may try to deceive others, whereas the malingerer consciously sets out to deceive others for his own ends and is under no illusions about what he is really doing.

   There is no rule for dealing with cases of this type; they have to be weighed up and dealt with individually.

Case 67   Female, aged 10

The record showed that this child had been emmetropic with acuities of R and L

6/6 +. Now, she said, her vision was blurred and she could only see at close distances. Refraction was difficult out of all proportion to the refractive error, but one must not be too ready to assume there is malingering in case some real pathological condition is missed:

R 6/12 + − 0.50DS 6/12 +
L 6/12 + − 0.50DS 6/12 +

Though she reported that vision seemed better with the above prescription, it did not really improve whatever lenses were tried. But on the other hand, it did not appreciably worsen if + 0.50DS was substituted for the − 0.50DS in the trial frame. Initially, she said she could not read any print on the near test card, but under pressure and encouragement she did pick out a few of the N 10 size words. As in the previous case, suspicions were aroused because this did not relate to the distance acuity.

It was decided to try the technique of positive assurance to resolve this problem. After a few changes of lenses which it was known would not result in any improvement, a pair of plano spheres were selected, and carefully set in the trial frame. She was again handed the reading chart. 'Now read this' she was told, the N 6 print being indicated. Unsuspectingly, she read on fluently. The planos were then removed, when immediately her poor vision returned and she was unable to continue!

It is unwise to prescribe glasses as a placebo in cases like this because it only serves to reinforce the deception. Instead she was confronted with the facts, and reassured that she could, indeed, see quite well, but her protestations persisted. Her parents could offer no reason for her behaviour so they were advised to talk it over sympathetically with the child, and to consult their GP if necessary.

But the deception ended uneventfully in a day or two. She was rechecked a month later, when her vision had returned to normal and the alleged symptoms had all disappeared.

(There are a wide variety of tests for malingering, and the optometrist should be prepared for such eventualities. There is an excellent chapter on this subject in Duke-Elder's *System of Ophthalmology*, Vol 5.)

As mentioned before, one must not be too ready to dismiss difficult refraction problems as due to malingering; there may be a genuine disorder that could easily be missed, as the next four cases illustrate.

Case 68   Female, aged 17   Accommodation and convergence weakness

This young lady complained of headaches after close work together with intermittent blurring of print. She was practically emmetropic:

R 6/6 + 0.25DS 6/6 +
L 6/6 + 0.25DS 6/6 +
3$^\Delta$ Esophoria Ortho V.   4$^\Delta$ Exophoria near vision.

In spite of the negligible refractive error, she was experiencing very real symptoms. Her convergence near point had receded to about 25 cm, and it transpired she had had occasional diplopia at near during the preceding few months. Accommodation was also weak, the near point varying around 20 cm. She was referred to her GP, but he thought that her symptoms were simply the aftermath of a prolonged illness, and requested that spectacles should be made up which would afford her some relief for the time being. Lenses were accordingly dispensed (with some misgivings) incorporating a weak reading addition and base-in prisms. Unfortunately the convergence defect increased rapidly, and only a short time later she was experiencing diplopia at all distances beyond 35 cm, rendering her glasses practically useless – a fact of which her family made sure the unfortunate practitioner was aware!

She was however then referred to a consultant, and after a long period her condition improved, and spectacles did then provide some benefit.

Case 69   Male, aged 14   Paralysis of accommodation

Close work had been 'going blurry' for the past week or two only. The pupils were large, but the reactions were normal.

R 6/9 + + 0.50DS 6/6 +
L 6/9 + + 0.50DS 6/6 +
1$^\Delta$ Esophoria Ortho. V distance Ortho. V and H near vision

One might have expected him to accept more plus, in view of the improvement in visual acuit with such a small correction, but this was not so. He said he was unable to read, and certainly he appeared to have no accommodation at all, although convergence was normal. With a plus reading addition, he could read easily, but only over a narrow range.

This did not resemble malingering, as the findings all fitted into a logical pattern. To make sure, he was again directed to the distance chart with R and L – 1.00DS in the trial frame. With these he was severely blurred, but the addition of a pair of + 1.00D spheres restored his vision to the original level. After referral it was explained that he had recently undergone a major operation, and it was considered that the weak accommodation was associated with general muscular fatigue. He was ordered a month's complete rest, following which the ocular symptoms largely subsided.

The next example is a cautionary tale which should be of interest to newcomers to the profession.

Case 70   Male, aged 12   Convergence weakness after trauma

This boy had been examined by another optometrist only six weeks previously because of frequent and persistent headaches, together with excessive fatigue and 'eyestrain' after close work. He had been given a thorough and careful examination, according to his parents, and had been told there was nothing wrong with his eyes and that glasses were not required. However, these symptoms persisted, so their GP was consulted, who advised them to seek another opinion. The eyes appeared quite healthy on examination, and he was practically emmetropic:

R $+0.25/-0.25$ 90 6/5
L -0.25 cyl 140 6/5
1^Δ Exophoria .Ortho V distance 4^Δ Exophoria near vision.

Accommodation was good and equal, but the convergence near point was well receded, fluctuating between about 22 and 30 cm; surprisingly, he had not complained of diplopia, but it was easily demonstrable within these distances. This was the one vital point that the previous examiner – a young and very conscientious individual – had overlooked. Possibly he had thought it unnecessary to check it as the near muscle balance was normal, which is a very common misconception.

Whatever the muscle balance findings are, and regardless of the means utilized to test them, the convergence near point does not *necessarily* relate to them and should always be checked separately. On questioning the parents, it was discovered that the child had been kicked on the head three or four months before, and they only now came to realize that his headaches and ocular symptoms must have commenced just afterwards. Spectacles should never be ordered without medical approval in cases like this, where there is a recent history of trauma, so he was referred. Some months later a report was received to the effect that after medical investigation and orthoptic treatment his convergence had reverted practically to normal.

Sometimes, of course, no explanation for poor vision can be found.

Case 71   Female, aged 15

As the only complaint was of difficulty in seeing the board at school it was expected that this would just be another routine refraction case:

R 6/12 $-0.25/-0.25$ 90 6/12
L 6/12 $+0.25$DS 6/12 +

Retinoscopy confirmed these findings. Ocular muscle balance was normal. Initially malingering was suspected, but the tests applied were all negative and her replies were perfectly consistent. All ophthalmic possibilities were explored without success; her eyes showed no abnormality at all, except that she simply could not achieve a normal standard of vision, so she was referred for a consultant's opinion. Extensive investigations were subsequently carried out, including e.e.g. and fluorescein angiography, but all proved negative. When last seen, 18 months after referral, nothing had been discovered which might account for the defective acuity.

It was impossible to judge whether she had always had poor vision, as she had not previously had a full eye examination, but it was reasonable to suppose that there must have been some deterioration as she had not made any complaint of visual difficulty before.

Occasionally, the reason for apparent difficulties in seeing can be so ludicrously simple that it can be overlooked by all concerned.

Case 72 Male, aged 19

This young man had failed his driving test. He had had his eyes rechecked by another optometrist only a month before, who had been unable to improve the acuity beyond 6/12. The patient consulted his doctor, who confirmed this low visual standard and referred him back to see if it was possible to make any improvement by modifying his prescription.

The optometrist concerned reported that this was the best that could be done but the GP, anxious to assist the patient, asked the writer to give a second opinion on the refraction and to see if any explanation for poor acuity could be found.

The refraction was:

R 6/15 $+4.75/-1.25 \times 150$ 6/12
L 6/15 $+4.50/-1.25 \times 50$ 6/12
12^Δ Esophoria Ortho. V distance

He was wearing a slightly weaker prescription, with which he could still read 6/12, but no better. He insisted that he could not read even N 12 size print with either pair. This inconsistency could not have been due to malingering, as he was obviously extremely keen to pass his driving test. A variety of tests were made in an attempt to identify the reasons for his difficulty, but without success. These were time-consuming and his appointment time became over-run to such an extent that I decided to see the next patient. Meanwhile he was left with my secretary who was instructed to see if she could encourage him to attempt the 6/9 line, and to see if he could pick out the N 6 type, which theoretically, should have been possible.

Not long after, however, she emerged with the explanation. 'He knows his letters,' she said, 'But he can't read!'

The reader may wonder how such a simple explanation had escaped two optometrists and a GP, but these things do occur. Obviously some of the blame rested with the patient, who had been too shy or too obtuse to admit his handicap. But on reflection, when he had said 'I can't read any of it', that was the unvarnished truth and we had not interpreted it literally enough.

This man did not require intensive investigation like the girl in Case 71 above, although the recorded acuity was the same. Perceptual processes and reading ability exert a considerable influence on letter acuity, and the illiterate individual cannot be expected to obtain 'normal vision' on standard letter charts.

Illiteracy, in general, indicates that the individual concerned is uninstructed or has been unable to develop the ability to read. At the other end of the scale we have people who have been able to read, but have lost the faculty, usually as a result of a cerebral lesion. The practitioner whose patients are mainly in the younger age groups will hardly ever see instances, but if his clientele consists predominantly of aged people he will inevitably encounter a number of cases. Unfortunately, owing to the very nature of their disorder, they may not realize how it has affected them, or well-meaning relatives bring them in and tell us that 'If only you could help (uncle/auntie/father, etc.) to read, it would give him something to do and it would be so much better for all of us'.

Case 73   Male, aged 63

This patient said that his vision had deteriorated, especially for reading, and mentioned that he had been having treatment for a cardiac disorder during the past five years. On previous visits he had been able to read 6/6 without difficulty, but it was certainly not so good now. The foveae were not well defined, but there were otherwise no significant signs in the fundi.

> R 6/36 $+0.50/-0.50\times$ V 6/18
> L 6/24 $+0.25/-0.50\times$ V 6/18
> 2^{Δ} Exophoria Ortho. V distance

He could not achieve better than 6/15 binocularly, but seemed less concerned about his low standard of vision than one would have expected. So far, refraction had been relatively straightforward, apart from the frustration of finding the acuity so persistently poor. But when reading tests were applied, it soon became evident that his visual problems were not entirely ocular in origin. He had been able to recognize inidividual letters adequately enough on the distance charts, but he was unable to combine them effectively except in the construction of a few of the simplest words.

Any hesitation during distance refraction had up to this stage been ascribed to his poor vision, but it was now found that attempts to improve reading by increasing the addition made no difference whatsoever. This handicap was therefore due to alexia and he could no longer interpret printed information of any sort. A field check demonstrated an almost complete R homonymous hemianopia with macular sparing (he had not been aware of this until the examination) indicating a left-sided cerebral lesion which tends to be associated with alexia.

It is usually best not to prescribe spectacles in cases like this, unless there is a sizeable distance error. Apparent improvement in acuity with a very small correction such as the above is often spurious – we push them a little harder in testing if vision seems poor, and they then try just that bit more!

Part of the art of prescribing, it should be evident, consists in knowing when not to prescribe. The patient who brings in a handbag full of old spectacles 'none of which are any good' is a daunting prospect and one must ask oneself frankly if it is really conceivable that not one of these previous prescribers has been able to understand her visual problems and provide a solution. Can you expect to succeed where so many others have failed?

The answer, of course, is 'Probably, no'. There are usually psychological reasons why such patients can never obtain satisfaction, but one should always try, as very rarely a genuine explanation for the difficulty may be found. But unless there is a really significant change in prescription, it is best to leave well alone. Similarly, if visual acuity is extremely poor, especially with aged patients, small changes are unwarranted. If there is a demonstrable improvement – so that the patient can now read, say, N 6 instead of N 8 at best – then the lenses should be replaced. Be careful, however, that in achieving this you have not increased the reading addition so much that the patient objects to having to hold print so close in.

Often the acuity is so poor in this group of cases that changes of as much as + 1.00DS or – 1.00DS make no perceptible difference. Many examples could be given but one will suffice to illustrate this point.

Case 74   Female, aged 84

Generalized hazing of the media, together with many lens opacities, were present, as is so common at this advanced age. She was wearing:

$$R \ +0.75/-0.75 \times 95 \ 1^{\Delta} \ \text{Base in}$$
$$L \ +0.75/-1.50 \times 5 \ 1^{\Delta} \ \text{Base in} \qquad \text{Add} \ +3.50 \ \text{reading}$$

Retinoscopy results were difficult to interpret because of the condition of the media, but seemed to suggest a low plus prescription with vertical minus cylinders. Careful and protracted subjective refraction, however, appeared to leave no doubt that concave spheres were required:

$$R \ 6/60 \ -0.50/-1.25 \times 90 \ 6/24$$
$$L \ 6/60 \ -0.25/-1.25 \times 90 \ 6/24 \ \text{partly} \qquad \text{Add} \ +4.00 \ \text{reading}$$

One must never be too confident about making improvements with acuities as low as this, and if there is the least doubt the patient should be shown what the effect of the alteration would be by putting trial lenses to make the appropriate difference in front of their existing spectacles, *and given time to consider it.*

In this case the patient could see exactly the same letters with either the new or the old prescription – the vast change in the left cylinder axis notwithstanding – so there was no point in altering the glasses. It may seem discouraging to find that one's best efforts have been to no avail, but it is much worse if one does not discover this until the patient calls to collect the glasses, and he repudiates them because 'I can see just as well with the old ones'.

Appendix 1
Revision Questions

1 What do the following notes on a patient's record signify? 'c/o asth, post V.D.U. & hor. dip. D/V am 3/52' (See section 4.3)

2 Suggest four gradings for use when anterior chamber depth is estimated. (See section 5.6)

3 What is the first lens power which is likely to be used for ophthalmoscopy? (See section 6.1)

4 A disc should be regarded as 'suspicious' if the cup:disc ratio is greater than 0.x. What is 'x'? (See section 6.2 and Fig. 6.10)

5 What reflection factor might be the best compromise for a retinoscope? 10, 40, 60, or 50 per cent? (See section 10.1 and Figs 10.2 and 10.3)

6 What 'working distance sphere' power for retinoscopy did Carter propose in 1986? It was one of these, + 5.00, + 1.00, + 10.00, + 20.00. Also, why such a departure? (See section 10.3)

7 A keratometer is usually calibrated for a particular refractive index. Is it 1.300, 1.333, 1.3375, or 1.75333? (See section 10.4)

8 The next question but one is about the duochrome or bichromatic test. What do you think would be a suitable question? (See question 10)

9 The accommodation induced by convergence is usually 1D per metre angle, up to 30 years of age. Does the ratio change after this? (See section 12.2)

10 What pair of maxima are recommended for the 'effective' transmission relative to tungsten light for bichromatic filters? It is one of these; 555 nm and 570 nm; 450 nm and 750 nm; 539 nm and 620 nm; 555 nm and 655 nm. (See section 11.1)

11 Does an alteration in vertex distance of a spectacle lens influence the near vision astigmatism measured in the spectacle plane? (See section 11.3)

12 Are many full-term babies highly astigmatic? (See section 13.2)

13 An object is 0.01 cm in size and is viewed at 33.3 cm. What visual angle would this subtend in prism dioptres and how is that related to near vision visual acuity expressed as an 'N' number? (See section 14.2)

14 Is senile myopia expected to appear before or after senile hyperopia? (See section 13.3)

15 Using a 'size lens' you magnify your right retinal image by 7 per cent and view a TV screen 50 cm directly in front of you. Describe the likely apparent tilt of the screen when viewed binocularly. If you close one eye would the apparent tilt alter? (See section 14.5 and Fig. 14.4)

16 How would you attempt to use prisms to catch a malingerer who claims that one eye (which is actually perfect) is virtually blind? (See section 15.1)

17 What extra methods could you prepare to use if you know that a deaf patient is booked for eye examination and refraction? Make a list of the points you should remember when communicating with the deaf. (See section 15.2)

18 What is the difference between 'moderating' and 'test' lenses in the 'immediate contrast' method? (See section 11.2)

19 In a bent form spectacle lens with a back surface power of $-6.00D$ what extra magnification is gained by increasing the thickness of the lens by 5 mm? (See section 14.5)

20 If a patient is hardly attending to what he is looking at during the early stages of dynamic retinoscopy, would you expect a 'with' movement rather than an 'against' movement? (See section 12.2)

Appendix 2
Test Yourself on Test Charts Standards

British Standard 4274:1968 gives basic requirements for test charts. You should be able to answer most of the following questions.

1. Which characters are to be in a frame 5 units high and 4 units wide and which should be in a frame 5 by 5 units?
2. The letters to be used are restricted to ten, which include the following D, E, N, P, R, U and Z, with three others. What are the three others?
3. What 'letter sizes' (distances in metres at which heights of letters subtend 5 minutes of arc) are included in a 'full chart'?
4. Which letter sizes may be omitted in an 'abridged' chart?
5. Do the letters have serifs?
6. What is the tolerance for the dimensions of a 6 metre letter?
7. To obviate discomfort glare the luminance of the immediate surround of the chart should not be below 30 per cent but as this may be unrealistic, what is the minumum per cent of the chart luminance, recommended for the immediate surround?
8. The desired minima should be greater by a certain percentage for new equipment, allowing for deterioration. What is this percentage?
9. State the desired minimum luminance for a new internally illuminated chart, in cd/square metre and the value for the illuminance level for a new externally illuminated chart, in lux.
10. What is the suggested 'uniformity ratio' for a chart, the ratio to the minimum to maximum luminance?

Answers
1. Letters, limited to D, E, F, H, N, P, R, U, V, Z, all 5 × 4; Broken rings and 'illiterate E' all 5 × 5.
2. F, H and V
3. 60, 36, 24, 18, 12, 9, 6, 5, 4, 3
4. 4 and 3
5. No
6. plus or minus 5 per cent

7 10 per cent
8 25 per cent
9 150 candelas per square metre and 600 lux
10 70 per cent

References and Select Bibliography

Adams T. (1968) The correction of aniseikonia: two case records. *The Optician*, **156**, 417–418

Adamson J. & Fincham E. F. (1939) Visual tolerances and their effect on the measurement of refraction, *Refractionist*, 405–411

Ardern, F. W. (1951) Some instruments used in refraction. Brit. J. Physiol, Opt. **8**, 1–42.

Aslin, R. N. (1987) The accommodative response system. In Salapatek, P. & Cohen, L. *Handbook of Infant Perception I.*, Academic Press, Orlando, pp. 44–60,

Association of Optometrists (undated) What is an eye examination? Association of Optometrists, London.

Banks M. S. (1980) Infant refraction and accommodation, *Int. Ophthal. Clinics*, **20**, 205–32.

Bannon R. E. (1947) The use of cycloplegics in refraction. *Amer. J. Optom. Arch. Amer. Acad. Optom.* **24**, 513–38.

Barratt C. D (1945) Sources of error and working methods in retinoscopy. *Brit. J. Physiol. Opt.* **5**, 35–40.

Bartlett J. D. & Jaanus S. D. (1989) *Clinical Ocular Pharmacology*, Butterworths, Boston.

Bennett A. G. (1960) Trial lenses ancient and modern. *Ophthalmic Optician*, **6**, 964–7, 1011–14, 1061–6.

Bennett A. G. (1963) The theory of bichromatic test. *Optician*, **146**, 291–6.

Bennett A. G. (1965) Ophthalmic test types. *Brit. J. Physiol. Opt.* **22**, 238–71

Bennett A. G. (1971) The near optical centration of invisible bifocals, Part 1. Spherical lenses, Part 2. Astigmatic lenses. *Optician*, **162**, 16–18. 8–10 in number 4202.

Bennett A. G. & Rabbetts R. B. (1984a) *Clinical Visual Optics*, Butterworths, London.

Bennett A. G. & Rabbetts R. B. (1984b) *Clinical Visual Optics*, Butterworths, London, pp. 303 & 367.

Borish I. M. (1970) *Clinical Refraction*, Professional Press, Chicago. pp. 5–133.

Borish I. M. (1975) *Clinical Refraction*, Professional Press, Chicago.

Bourque L. B., Cosand B. B., Drews C., Waring G. O., Lynn. M. & Cartwright C. (1986) Reported satisfaction, fluctuation of vision and glare, among patients one year after surgery in the Prospective Evaluation of Radial Keratotomy (PERK) Study. *Arch. Ophthal.* **104**, 356–63.

British College of Optometrists (undated) *Guidelines for Candidates, Supervisors, and Examiners on the Professional Qualifying Examination.*

British College of Optometrists (undated) *Code of Ethics and Guidelines.*

Carter J. H. (1986) A system of retinoscopy for the aged eyes. *Amer. J. Optom., Physiol. Opt.* **63**, 298–9.

Cashell Y. & Durran I. (1974) *Handbook of Orthoptic Principles*, Churchill Livingstone, London.

Chawla H. (1983) *Essential Ophthalmology*, Churchill Livingstone, London.

Charman W. N. (1975) Some sources of discrepancy between static retinoscopy and subjective refraction. *Brit. J Physiol. Opt.*, **30**, 108–18

Charman W. N. & Jennings J. A. M. (1974) Evaluation of laser refraction using naive subjects. *Ophthal. Opt.*, **14**, 1041–4.

Cholerton M. (1948) *Some Aspects of Oculo Refractive Technique*, Hammond, London.

Classé J. G. (1989) *Legal Aspects of Optometry*, Butterworths, Boston.

Cockburn D. M. (1987) Why patients complain about their new spectacles. *Clin. Exp. Optom.* **70**, 91–5.

Cole J. (1945) Developments in infinity balance technique. *Refractionist*, **32**, 195–9

Cooper J. (1987) Accommodative dysfunction. In *Diagnosis and Management in Vision Care*, (Ed. by J. P. Amos) Butterworth Scientific, London, pp. 431–54.

Davies L. M. *et al.* (1986) A cost-effective comparison of the intraocular lens and the contact lens in aphakia. *Trans. Ophthal. Soc. UK.*, **105**, 304–13.

Draper I. (1980) *Lecture Notes on Neurology*, 5th Edn. Blackwell Scientific Publications, Oxford.

Duke-Elder W. S. (1970) *System of Ophthalmology*, **V**, 487–501. Kimpton, London.

Dunscombe K. O. (1933) A new and remarkably sensitive test for astigmatism. *Brit. J. Physiol. Opt.* **7**, 112–28.

Emsley H. H. (1963) The keratometer: measurement of concave surfaces. *Optician* **146**, 161–8.

Emsley H. H. (1973) *Visual Optics*, Vols 1 & 2, (5th edn) Butterworths, London.

Fahle M. & Mohn G. (1989) Assessment of visual function in suspected ocular malingering. *Brit. J. Ophthal.* **73**, 651–4.

Fletcher R. (1946) Presbyopic additions, a survey of 300 cases. *Optician*, **III**, 246–52

Fletcher R. J. (1951–1952) Astigmatic accommodation. *Brit. J. Physiol. Opt.*, **8**, 73–94; 129–160; 193–224; 8–32.

Fletcher R. (1954a) *Aspects of Intro-Ocular Physiology*. Hatton Press, London.

Fletcher R. (1954b) Near vision astigmatism. *Optician*. **127**, 341–50.

Fletcher R. (1955) The ophthalmometer in contact lens fitting. *Brit. J. Physiol. Opt.*, **12**, 37–9.

Fletcher R. J. (1960) Instruments used for objective examination. In *The principles and practice of refraction* (Ed. by G. H. Giles) Hammond, London, pp. 595–616.

Fletcher R. (1961) *Ophthalmics in Industry*, Hatton Press, London.

Fletcher R. & Voke J. (1985) *Defective Colour Vision*, Hilger, Bristol.

Freeman H. & Hodd F. A. B (1955) Comparative analysis of retinoscopic and subjective refraction. *Brit. J. Physiol. Opt.* **12**, 8–36.

Giles G. H. (1960) *The Principles and Practice of Refraction*, Hammond, London.

Gross D. A. & Eskridge J. B. (1987) Myopia. In *Diagnosis and Management in Version Care* (Ed. by J. F. Amos) Butterworths, Boston, pp. 142–55.

Griffiths, G. (1988) Autorefractors – their use and usefulness. *Optician*, **196**, 22–9.

Grolman B. (1966) Binocular refraction – a new system. *New England J. Optom*, **17**, 118–29.

Guillon M. L. (1978) *A study of objective refraction devices in abnormal eyes*. Ph. D. thesis, The City University , London.

Hawkeswell A. (1975) The development of a portable space eikonometer. *Brit. J. Physiol. Opt.* **30**, 25–33.

Henson D. B. (1983) *Optometric instrumentation*. Butterworths, London, pp. 179–83

Hirsch M. J. (1960) Refractive changes with age. In *Vision of the aging patient*, (Ed. by M. J. Hirsch & R. E Wick) Chilton, Philadelphia. pp. 63–82.

Hodd F. A. B. (1951) The measurement of spherical refraction by retinoscopy. *Trans. Int. Opt. Cong.* BOA, London, 191–231.

Horgen G., Aaras A., Fagerthun H. E. & Larsen S. E. (1989) The work posture and the postural load of the neck/shoulder muscles when correcting presbyopia with different types of multifocal lenses on VDU workers, Paper to International Conference on Work with Display Units (2) Boston.

Humphriss D. & Woodruff E. W. (1962) Refraction by immediate contrast. *Brit. J. Physiol Opt.* **19**, 15–20.

Kanski J. (1986) *The Eye in Systemic Disease,* Butterworths, London.

Kramer K. K., Francis G. L. & Appleton B. (1979) Ocular malingering and hysteria: diagnosis and management. *Surv. Ophthal.,* **24**, 89–96.

Kritzinger E. E. & Beaumont H. M. (1987) *A Colour Atlas of Optic Disc Abnormalities,* Wolfe Medical, London.

Layton A., Dickinson J. & Pluznick M. (1978) Perception of blur in optometric tests. *Amer. J. Optom. Physiol. Opt.,* **55**, 75–7.

Larke J. (1985) *The Eye in Contact Lens Wear,* Butterworths, London.

Mets M. B. (1988) Drops, drops, drops in pedriatric opthalmology. In *Year Book of Ophthalmology 1988,* (Ed. by J. T. Ernest, & T. A. Deutsch.) Chicago, Year Book Medical Pub., 17–20.

McCaghrey, G. (1989) Autorefractors, friend or foe. *Optom. Today,* 30 June 6–9.

McMinn R., Hitchings R. & Logan B. (1981) *A Colour Atlas of Head and Neck Anatomy,* Wolfe Medical, London.

Michaels D. D. (1985) *Visual Optics and Refraction,* Blackwell, Oxford.

Michelson J. B. (1984) *A Colour Atlas of Uveitis Diagnosis,* Wolfe Medical, London.

Miller D. & Stegmann R. (1987) Approaches to protection against light-induced changes in the eye. In *Clinical Light Damage to the Eye.* (Ed. by D. Miller), Springer, New York, pp. 165–79.

Millidot M. & Millodot S. (1989) Presbyopia correction and the accommodation in reserve. *Ophthal, Physiol. Opt.* **9**, 126–32.

Mohindra I. (1975) A technique for infant visual examination. *Amer. J. Optom.,* **52**, 867–70.

Mohrman R. C. & Hogan J. G. (1977) Automatic retinoscopy: the Ophthalmetron. *Optician,* **173**, 20–29.

Molteno A. C. B. & Molteno T. E. S. (1977) A new system of refraction for use by the general practitioner. *S. Afr. Med. J.* **52**, 354–355.

Morgan M. W. (1960) Accommodative changes in presbyopia and their correction. In *Vision of the aging patient.* (Ed. by M. J. Hirsch & R. E. Wick) Chilton, Philadelphia, pp. 83–145.

North R, & Henson D. B. (1985) Adaption to lens-induced heterophorias. *Amer. J. Physiol. Opt.* **62**, 774–80.

Nyak B. H., Ghose S. & Singh J. P. (1987) A comparison of cycloplegic and manifest refractions on NR-1000F. *Brit. J. Ophthal.* **87**, 73–5.

O'Connor Davies P. H., Hopkins G. A. & Pearson R. M. (1989) *The Actions and Uses of Ophthalmic Drugs,* Butterworths, London.

Olson M. (1987) Early intervention for children with visual impairment. In The effectiveness of early intervention for at-risk and handicapped children, (Ed. by M. J. Guralnick & F. C. Bennett) Academic Press, Orlando. pp. 297–324.

Pascal J. I. (1952) *Studies in Visual Optics,* Mosby, St Louis.

Pickwell D. (1984) *Binocular Vision Anomalies,* Butterworths, London.

Rabbetts R. B. & Bennett A. G. (1986) Near vision effective power losses in trial and prescription lenses. *Optometry Today,* **26**, 14–19, 36–38.

Raubitscheck E. (1952) The Raubitscheck arrow test for astigmatism. *Amer. J. Ophthal.,* **35**, 1331–9.

Reading V. M. & Weale R. A. (1974) Macular pigment and chromatic aberration. *J. Opt. Soc. Amer.,* **64**, 231–4.

Reeves B. (1989) The accommotrac vision trainer. *Optician,* **198**, 17–20.

Remole A. (1989) Anisophoria and anisoeikonia. Part. 1, the relation between optical anisophoria and anisoeikonia. *Optom. & Vision Science,* **66**, 659–70.

Ryan V. (1975) Predicting aniseikonia in anisometropia. *Amer. J. Optom. Physiol. Opt.,* **52**, 96–105.

Safir, A *et al.* (1970) Studies in refraction, 1. The precision of retinoscopy. *Arch. Ophthal.* **84**, 49–61.

Sletteberg O., Bertlesen T. & Høvding G. (1989) The prognosis of patients with hysterical visual impairment. *Acta. Ophthal.* **67**, 159–63.

Spalton D., Hitchings R. & Hunter P. (1984) *Atlas of Clinical Ophthalmology,* Churchill Livingstone, London.

Spooner J. (1969) *Ocular Anatomy,* Hatton Press, London.

Stark L. (1988) Presbyopia in light of accommodation. *Amer. J. Optom. Physiol. Opt.* **65**, 407–16.

Swaine W. (1925) The relation of visual acuity and accommodation to ametropia. *Trans. Opt. Soc.,* **27**, 9–27.

Taylor S. (1939) Dynamic retinoscopy. *Brit. J. Physiol. Opt.* **13**, 110–30.

Taylor G. & Austen D. (1986) *Law and Management in Optometric Practice,* Butterworths, London.

Vale J. & Cox B. (1985) *Drugs and the Eye,* Butterworths, London.

Wagstaff D. F. (1966) The objective measurement of the amplitude of accommodation. *Optician,* **151**, 105–9.

Walls G. L. (1942) *The Vertebrate Eye,* Cranbrook Inst. Sci., Bloomfield Hills.

Weale R. A. (1963) *The Aging Eye,* Lewis, London.

Weale R. A (1989) Presbyopia toward the end of the 20th century. *Surv. Opthal.* **34**, pp. 15–30.

Wilkinson J. D., Shaw S. & Fenton D. A. (1987) *Dermatology,* Churchill Livingstone, London.

Wolff E. (Rev. by R. H. Last) (1968) *Anatomy of The Eye and Orbit,* Lewis, London.

Wray L. (1971) Some errors in prescribing. *Optician,* **161**, 12–20.

Young F. A *et al.* (1971) Comparison of cycloplegia and non-cycloplegic refractions of eskimos. *Amer. J. Optom. Arch. Amer. Acad. Optom.,* **48**, 814–25.

Zetterström C. (1985) A cross over study of the cycloplegic effects of a single topical application of Cyclopentolate-Phenylephrine and routine atropinization for 3.5 days. *Acta Ophthal.,* **63**, 525–9.

Index